TAKE
CONTROL
OF YOUR
HEALTH

BOOKS BY DR. MERCOLA

No Grain Diet

Dr. Mercola's Total Health

Bird Flu Hoax

Sweet Deception

TAKE CONTROL OF YOUR HEALTH

Dr. Joseph Mercola

with

Dr. Kendra Degen Pearsall

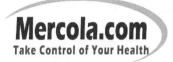

Mercola.com
Take Control of Your Health

TAKE CONTROL OF YOUR HEALTH
By Dr. Joseph Mercola and Dr. Kendra Pearsall

Publisher: Mercola.com
1443 West Schaumburg Rd.
Schaumburg, IL 60194

This book may be bulk ordered at special rates.
Contact customerservice@mercola.com or write to
Mercola.com, 1443 West Schaumburg Road, Schaumburg, IL 60194

Printed in the United States of America   First Edition

Contents

FOREWORD

Dr. Mercola is one of very few physicians who combine a long-term view of diet and human health with individualized diet recommendations. He's one of even fewer who help his patients improve their health and prevent disease by combining diet principles with attention to emotions and body energies. If you haven't read anything by Dr. Mercola before, you'll get excellent advice in this book, but I also recommend you visit his website, www.Mercola.com. You'll learn much, much more about getting well and staying well!

About that very-long-term view that Dr. Mercola takes: When I was a pre-medical student in the 1960s (according to my children, the "Dark Ages"), I took the same courses in biology, chemistry, biochemistry, and physics that all the other "pre-meds" did. But I also "majored" in anthropology, because I thought that if I was going to try to take care of people's health, I'd best learn as much about us people as I possibly could.

I learned that the very first remains of any kind of people at all date back approximately 2 million years, and that the remains of people who appear to be the same as we, date back many thousands of years. I also learned that for all those years, what our ancestors ate were various parts of animals, fish, shellfish, the occasional egg stolen from a bird's nest, vegetables, roots, nuts, fruits and berries for a month or two a year, and insects (that's still done in Australia). But until approximately *500 generations ago*, when various groups slowly "invented" agriculture and domesticated animals, *absolutely no one* ate grains, and no one at all drank milk or ate any other dairy products! (Can you imagine a pre-historic cow holding still to be milked? Prehistoric cattle ran away from us humans as fast as they could!).

I took some history classes too and learned that only four to five hundred years ago, refined sugar was as expensive as gold. Only kings, queens, and the very wealthy could afford very tiny quantities. Before that, no one had any at all! We learned that synthetic, artificial food chemicals, flavors, and preservatives were just invented in the 19th century, as well as margarine. Prior to that time, no one ate any of these "foods" at all!

However, my biochemistry classes taught me that it's very likely that our 21st century human biochemistry has worked exactly the same (or incredibly close) for *many thousands of generations.*

What does a human biochemical system do? It manages the molecules and atoms of material reality that helps keep us alive. It just makes sense that if our personal biochemistries are exactly the same as human biochemistry has been for all that time, we'll stay healthier if we use the same materials (food and drink) to "fuel" that biochemistry that our ancestors have used for thousands of years. And if we can't duplicate those ancestral diets exactly, we should come as close as we possibly can.

Here's an (admittedly satirical) way of making the same point, from the first book I published (*Dr. Wrights Book of Nutritional Therapy*, 1979):

> *The hunter stalked his prey through the awakening forest. As the early rays of the sun filtered through the branches overhead, he moved noiselessly from tree to tree. Finally halting, he quickly but carefully fitted an arrow to his bowstring, aimed, and let fly. This time he hit his mark; he was glad, because he had not eaten since the previous day. He walked to where his arrow had fallen, carefully removed the*

chocolate-covered jelly doughnut, and walked away, eating his breakfast.

The four women had wandered far to find food for the midday meal. Finally the oldest, wise in the ways of their tribe, saw a familiar plant. She'd only seen it once as a girl, but had remembered. From it they gathered the cans of spaghetti and meatballs, and started home.

The children, thirsty again, ran to a tree they knew well. At this time of year, it provided the most delicious orange-flavored fruit drink, with 50% more vitamin C than the competing tree on the other side of their encampment.

Never happened, did it? And we shouldn't be eating that stuff, or anything else like it! And that's the very-long-term view that Dr. Mercola takes about diet and health.

Although our general human biochemical patterns have been the same for all those years, we are all uniquely created with our own individual variations on the general human pattern. While individualization is what Dr. Mercola (and any good physician) does with each client he or she sees in person, individualization can't be done nearly as well by a book. However, he makes a good start by helping you to apply the principles of *Nutritional Typing,* which helps to group our individual biochemistries into several general patterns.

If you're not feeling well and follow Dr. Mercola's advice, your health will improve! If you have no health problems, and don't want any, following Dr. Mercola's advice will keep most illness away.

—Jonathan V. Wright, M.D.
Tahoma Clinic, Renton, Washington
www.tahoma-clinic.com
Author (with Lane Lenard, Ph.D.) of
Why Stomach Acid Is Good For You (2001)
Maximize Your Vitality and Potency for Men Over 40 (1999)
Natural Hormone Replacement for Women Over 45 (1997)

FOREWORD

Dr. Mercola is at the forefront of a health revolution that will change the face of our nation. With obesity, cancer, and heart disease at an all-time high and the incidence of digestive and immune-related disorders increasing by the moment, the time to change is now. I have known Dr. Mercola for over four years, and out of the thousands of physicians I speak to each year, he stands out as one of the most committed, driven, and insightful health practitioners today. Our mutual reverence for the timeless health truths set in motion at the creation of time has made us "kindred spirits" on a mission that is beyond even the scope of our imagination. His commitment to finding the highest quality solutions for his patients' health is second to none.

Always willing to step outside of the proverbial "box," Dr. Mercola is never satisfied with status quo; despite the nearly miraculous results he achieves with his patients on a daily basis, he is always looking to refine and improve his protocols. Through his ground-breaking website and e-newsletter—that, incidentally, is read by hundreds of thousands each week—Dr. Mercola gives all of us commonsense truths, backed by history and science, that can make an immediate impact on our health, if we take action. His most important written work yet, *Take Control Of Your Health,* uses the wisdom gleaned from reading thousands of studies. More importantly, however, is that this program has succeeded in helping thousands of patients overcome seemingly incurable ailments. Through his book, Dr. Mercola leads us to a practical health plan that truly works.

Take Control Of Your Health provides the reader with a proven program for optimizing weight, energy, and health by eating properly according to one's specific biochemistry. The reader will learn about all the "right" and "wrong" foods and how they can affect the quest for optimal health—physically and emotionally. By ignoring the notion of "politically correct nutrition," Dr. Mercola's new book gives us the following cutting-edge health information:

- Essential steps to health and optimal weight that you need to know.

- The major ways artificial sweeteners can cause serious health problems and how to avoid the risks.

- The high-sugar culprits (disguised by food manufacturers as "healthy") that are actually contributors to obesity and a variety of diseases in children and adults.

- How pasteurization destroys the health value of milk and what alternatives you have.

- Why sleep is one of the most important keys to health and the most effective ways to sleep well.

- Why red meat and eggs may actually be health foods and how to ensure you're consuming the right kind.

- The fat that can actually help you stay thin, improve your metabolism, and improve your immune system.

That's only the beginning; those are just a *few* of the groundbreaking health secrets you will learn from reading and using this book. Dr. Mercola's *Take Control Of Your Health* is not a book to read once and put on your shelf to collect dust; it is meant to be used every day as a guidebook while you are on the road to optimal health.

Let me be the *first* to congratulate you on making today the first day of the rest of your health!

God Bless You,

—Jordan S. Rubin,
Author of *The Maker's Diet*

INTRODUCTION
How This Program Changes Peoples' Lives

You are likely reading this book because you have become progressively frustrated with the traditional medical model which relies on expensive drugs and surgeries and in no way, shape, or form treat the underlying cause of disease. While this model works well for acute traumas, it is an unmitigated disaster for the chronic degenerative diseases that are your major risk of death and disability.

You are likely fed up with the trillions of dollars being spent every year in the current model that results in the premature death and disability of millions while enriching multinational drug corporations.

Fortunately, there is hope. By adopting the time tested principles of natural living you can start to Take Control of Your Health. For the last three decades I have been committed to learning and applying these principles and have helped hundreds of thousands of people through my practice just outside of Chicago and my website.

The message is clear. With some coaching and encouragement you can achieve health independence and you don't have to rely on the drug model for answers to your health care challenges.

I have chose to include the following stories from a few of my patients and subscribers to illustrate how following the natural health principles in this book can transform your health. Although these patient letters may sound incredible, their results are typical of what we see when our patients implement the program.

Lost 20 Pounds and Gained Amazing Energy

The Take Control of Your Health Program from Dr. Mercola, as well as his newsletters have dramatically changed my life. Before putting into practice these basic beginning principles, I was over-weight, carrying extra pounds from my pregnancies. I was borderline diabetic and miserable with myself, as well as having poor health and no energy.

About a month and a half ago I began focusing on changing my behaviors as well as what I put into my body. In that short amount of time, I have lost 20 pounds and have gained some amazing energy. I can finally play with my children longer and [am] continuing to see benefits that I didn't know were possible.

I have always had trouble with sinus infections and colds and those have dramatically decreased in severity and frequency. I look forward to continued health improvements and weight stabilization as I continue implementing these life-changing steps. I recommend everyone find their true nutritional type and see what it can do for you.

—*M. Roeder, Rambleridge, Nebraska* ✑

Overcame Diabetes

I decided to visit Dr. Mercola in Chicago after I had learned about his nutritional typing technique. I am a diabetic and until three months ago, I was at the point in my life where I can truly say that I was on my deathbed. I had absolutely no energy to get myself out of bed in the morning to get to work, and on the days I had off, I stayed in bed. I was overweight and on 16 medications for diabetes and high blood pressure. The state of health that I was in was causing me to lose my job and my life.

Dr. Mercola educated me about his Take Control of Your Health program, which includes limited grains, and nutritional typing . . . I started to follow the nutritional typing food recommendations for the mixed type and realized it wasn't as hard as I thought it was going to be. I created a meal plan to follow and used it for my nutritional type. I eliminated grains and sugars and added a lot of green vegetables to my diet, such as spinach and turnip greens. I also eliminated 98 percent of all breads and most potatoes.

What helped me the most in the beginning was EFT. By far, EFT has been one of the most helpful tools for me. The method did appear strange to me at first but by using the technique it helped me overcome my food cravings and helped me focus on my job. EFT gave me the self-determination to feel better and conquer my health problems. I set goals for myself and visualized every one of them and set out to accomplish them. I also prayed a lot.

It took me about three weeks till I noticed a difference in myself, and within two months of being on Dr. Mercola's program I lost 11 pounds and through nutritional typing I lowered my blood sugar. And the best news is, I am only on six medications, as opposed to 16, and I am working with Dr. Mercola to eliminate the rest of them . . .

By following Dr. Mercola's plan, I have more energy than I have ever had before. When I first saw him I wasn't exercising and now I enjoy walking two to three miles a day, three to five times a week. I feel so much better about myself. I can finally say that I am on my way to becoming independently healthy.

—*Harrel Hill, Tupelo, Mississippi* ❧

Take Control of Your Health Program Heals a Family

In about one year, the Take Control of Your Health Program . . . has helped my mildly autistic nine-year-old, my child with apraxia and severe phoenetical speech disorder, my attention deficit hyperactivity disorder first grader and second grader with depression tendencies.

You won't believe how much it helped me . . . I was in constant pain and just didn't know it because it was with me since I was in grade school. Obsessive-compulsive disorder tendencies, depression, severe anxiety, severe back pain, chronic fatigue, whatever, you name it, I had it. And now it's gone. My nonverbal learning disorder hubby is getting better, slowly, but surely. I have known for six years all this was related to diet, because I felt it in my gut! But now *I know*, and I want to spread the word.

I was searching like crazy (and my family had been on every kind of diet around), and six years later, I've found it. The final last thing I cut out was wheat. It had a major impact on my back pain ... It's all about listening to the body, being honest and doing the right thing . . . It can't get any better than this, and if you follow Dr. Mercola's Take Control of Your Health Program, food simply tastes better, and eating is more fun & relaxed!

—*Carolyn Wilcoxon, Cedar Rapids, Iowa* ॐ

At Age 29, I Thought I Was Going to Die

At age 29, I thought I might die. After visiting over 30 different medical doctors for treatment of an endless list of health problems that "traditional" medicine simply did not cure, I felt I could not handle any more illness. Just some of my health problems included: fibromyalgia, chronic fatigue syndrome, repeated bacterial infections, severe asthma, a tumor on my head, thyroid disease, recurrent bouts with the flu, skin cancer on my shoulder, hypothyroid, depression, severe joint pain.

On top of this, I visited rheumatologists, gastroenterologist, otolarynologist, dermatologist, gynecologist and so on, much like a game of basketball, my "traditional" doctors would treat their one assigned area of the body and bounce me on to another "-ologist" to treat a different illness.

And yet, nobody could put the pieces together and figure out that something systemic was slowly killing me.

You can imagine my surprise when as a vegetarian Dr. Mercola informed me that I was a protein nutritional type and should eat meat. I fought this at first but as I grew sicker, I decided to give it a try.

I felt better almost immediately with the new diet and have followed it ever since.

Within six months of my implant removal, coupled with the change in lifestyle that I have made with the Optimal Wellness Center, my slow health improvements flew into hyper-speed and I am recovering!

The Optimal Wellness Center and Dr. Mercola's Take Control of Your Health Program is a place of truth, where the body is taught to heal and live healthy, where medical myths and hazards are exposed, where life is simplified and control given back to the patient to heal thyself.

—*Amy Pearlman, Lincolnshire, Illinois* ❧

Most health problems are a result of unhealthy lifestyle. Regrettably, rather than addressing health problems through education and understanding, our medical system gives people drugs to counteract their symptoms. The principles of the Take Control Of Your Health program are not "quick fixes" to superficially cover up your symptoms. Instead, they teach you how make natural lifestyle changes to restore and revitalize your body. You will be able to regain your health, and in some cases even reverse very serious diseases. You may also find you have increased energy, better sleep, and a brighter outlook on life.

"One of the first duties of the physician is to educate the masses not to take medicine."

—*Sir William Osler* (1849–1919), one of the greatest medical icons and frequently referred to as the Father of Modern Medicine. From *The Principles and Practice of Medicine* (1892)

CHAPTER:

Taking Control of Your Life

- Are you sick and tired of being sick and tired?
- Are you frustrated that, when you are sick, your doctor only prescribes you drugs?
- Do you feel a loss of power by having to rely on your doctor for all the answers to your health problems?
- Have you paid a fortune for your drugs or surgery, only to suffer many serious side effects?

The odds are high that you answered "yes" to one or more of these questions and are interested in taking back control of your health.

The goal of this book is to empower you with simple, practical insights and knowledge to becoming independently healthy without needing to rely on drugs, surgery, or doctors for anything but acute traumas. Much of this information has been suppressed by the media because it conflicts with the drugs supplied by the drug companies. Their interests are in direct conflict to you applying these effective and less expensive alternatives.

You may have been brought up to believe that your health depends exclusively on the quality of the healthcare you receive. The truth is, your health is your responsibility. You are the only person who can make the lifestyle decisions that contribute to your well being. You are the one who must take the steps to preserve your health and promote your wellness. Only you have the power to create wellness for yourself.

Your power lies in the choices you make every day on your own behalf. If you act out of habit or fixed attitudes, you may not be using your choices wisely to create wellness in your life. To create wellness you must expand your focus beyond mere physical health, and:

- Strive to balance and integrate your physical, emotional, and dietary choices

- Gather information and make informed wellness-oriented choices

- Actively participate in your health decisions and healing process

Achieving Health and Wellness Rather Than Treating Disease

According to the World Health Organization:

"Health is more than the absence of disease. Health is a state of optimal well-being."

Optimal well-being is a concept of health that goes beyond the curing of *illness* to one of achieving *wellness*. Achieving wellness requires balancing the various aspects of the whole person.

These aspects are physical, emotional, and dietary. This broader, holistic approach to health involves the integration of all of these aspects and is an ongoing process.

Obstacles to Wellness

I want you to start your path on this journey with open eyes, because you need to realize the cards are heavily stacked against you. There is a conflict of interest in the present system that practices fraud and deception when it comes to providing you with honest, reliable, and accurate information regarding your health.

Just look at the numbers. In 2006 the United States spent over two trillion dollars on "health" care. The majority of the money spent had absolutely nothing to do with health or health promotion, but everything to do with expensive drugs and surgeries designed to suppress symptoms of diseases.

Now, I have no problem investing trillions of dollars if the return on this massive investment showed improvement in health-care. But if you examine the numbers, it sure doesn't appear to be the case.

When compared with nearly two dozen other industrialized countries, the United States has the highest infant mortality rate and the lowest life expectancy for people who have reached age 60.

Fatally Flawed Conventional Paradigm

This is not a surprise, as the most common cause of death in America really isn't cancer or heart disease or accidents. It is the fatally flawed medical system that focuses on using toxic and expensive pharmaceutical band-aids that in no way, shape, or form treat the underlying cause of the disease.

There has been an enormous corporate infrastructure supporting this belief system, and the United States wastes well over two trillion dollars EVERY year on "heath care" that relies on expensive drugs and surgical solutions which rarely address the underlying cause of the problem. Now, $2 trillion dollars is a lot of money, but the more tragic costs are costs of human life: it bears repeating that the #1 cause of death in the United States is complications from drugs and surgery. Instead of saving us, our medical system is killing us.

Drug Companies Control The Health Care System— Not Your Doctor

Unless you're a part of the conventional medical system like I used to be, you may not realize that the multinational drug corporations control most of health care, including the medical education of doctors. Most physicians do not question this fact; they are unable to see the forest through the trees.

But let's examine the facts.

The largest political lobbying force in Washington is not the oil, tobacco, or gun lobby, but the drug companies. They have more lobbyists in Washington than there are congressmen. By wisely leveraging this force they have been able to manipulate legislation that highly favors their ability to sell their expensive band-aids.

Every year they spend over 4 billion dollars on direct-to-consumer advertising that is legal in only two countries in the world: the United States and New Zealand. Even the tobacco and alcohol industries haven't been able to pull this off.

If that weren't bad enough, drug companies spend over $16 billion to influence physicians' prescription habits. That is over $10,000 per year for every physician in the United States. There are dozens of carefully controlled studies which demonstrate that the perks doctors receive from the drug companies have a measurable effect on which drugs they prescribe. In fact, drug companies are able to monitor how many times a physician writes a prescription for their drugs and then bonus them accordingly.

All this investment has paid off, as in 2006, pharmacies filled nearly **5 billion prescriptions**; this is more than one prescription a month for every person in the United States

Confessions Of A Former Sugar Junkie

Many have wondered how I started my journey into natural health and became such a rebel when it comes to bucking the conventional medical system.

It has been my experience that most people start their journey into natural health from one of two paths. The most common way is that they develop a serious disease, and the conventional medical approach miserably fails them and they are forced to seek out alternative treatment options.

The other common entry into natural health is by growing up in a family that teaches natural health principles. That was not my case at all.

I am the first born son and the oldest of five children. Childhood was difficult for me at times. Formal education for my parents ended before either one of them graduated from high school. As far back as I can remember, they each worked day and night at more than one job to feed our

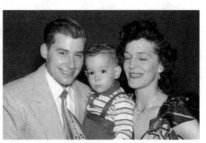

Me at age two with my parents Tom and Jeanette

family of seven. I also worked at odd jobs starting in junior high, in order to have the money I needed for bus fare and lunch at school. My parents were gone much of the time. One "consolation" for me was a never ending supply of sugary snacks that were at my disposal. Twinkies, Ding-Dongs, Pop-Tarts and various sugary cereals lined the cupboards at our house. My siblings and I indulged deeply and frequently in these palate-pleasers. By the time I reached college, I paid a price for this. I had a mouthful of dangerous mercury fillings from all my cavities, and severe cystic acne.

I have no idea why I was inspired to health and wellness; it makes absolutely no sense to me. There simply wasn't anything in my environment to encourage it. However, my mom helped create in me a passionate desire to read and to learn. Before I knew it, one book lead to another, and eventually to a book on health.

My First Steps On The Road Less Traveled

One of the books I read when I was 14 years old was written by Dr. Ken Cooper, the physician in charge of training astronauts to get in shape. He was a colonel in the U.S. Air Force who retired and went into private practice and built his fitness center outside of Dallas.

I read his first book in 1968 and was inspired to get fit. I chose running as my exercise. Today it is not uncommon to find major races that approach 50,000 runners participating. But I can assure you that in 1968 there were barely that many people in the entire United States that were running. It was an activity primarily restricted to school competitions.

When I started running on the streets in my inner city Chicago neighborhood, older kids would jeer at me and throw rocks and bottles, and many older adults believed I was running away from the scene of a crime.

I persisted in spite of the challenge and have continued to exercise and run for nearly forty years now. This was not only the beginning of my journey into natural health but also into challenging conventionally-held health beliefs.

You may not know this, but in the late '60s, a majority of physicians thought running and exercise actually CAUSED heart disease. If a person had a heart attack, they were prescribed weeks or months of strict bed rest or inactivity so their heart could "recover" and not be stressed.

Like many traditionally held health beliefs today, nothing could be farther from the truth. I have spent the last four decades learning more about health and continuing to challenge the norm. It seems the information I've advocated—once labeled as quackery by so-called experts—is now accepted as fact.

A Love Affair With Prescription Drugs

For all of high school and a good part of college, I worked as a pharmacy apprentice in a medical clinic with about eight physicians. In that environment, I developed the erroneous belief that drugs had the power to heal all sickness, and this belief influenced my desire to become a physician.

I eventually got into medical school in 1978 and did a three-year family medicine residency program in Chicago from 1982–1985.

I believe, largely as a result of my pharmacy apprentice training, I graduated medical school as a major drug-prescribing physician. I must have put thousands of people on antidepressants, because nearly everyone I saw was depressed.

It got to be so bad that the associate pastor of the church I attended at the time (one of the largest in the country) called me. Over half of his staff was on antidepressants that I prescribed. I realized then that perhaps something was amiss with this way of treating depression, and it spurred my interest to research other alternatives to drugs.

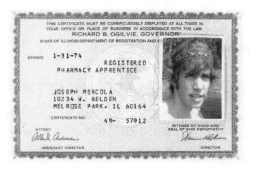

Back in 1973, I went from a hippie to a brainwashed drug promoting pharmacy apprentice.

My Transition To Natural Health

I had read Dr. Crook's book, *The Yeast Connection*, shortly after I finished my residency program. His premise was that yeast caused a variety of common diseases. His theory seemed plausible, so I tried to work with it. Unfortunately I disregarded his diet recommendations and went straight for prescribing antifungal drugs. Needless to say it did not work, and I completely discounted his work.

It took me another seven years before I reexamined his approach. As a result of caring for some patients with challenging health conditions who were simply not improving with conventional methods, I determined that yeast was a part of the problem. This time I was a bit wiser and used his diet, which consisted of a rigid sugar restriction. Lo and behold it worked! His book had a list of physicians who were using the program, and I found a local mentor, Dr. Gary Oberg, who guided me into a network of physicians who understood health at a deeper level.

From there I attended weekend seminars all over the country once or twice a month. This, combined with reading and listening to audio programs, helped me gain an understanding of using natural medicine to treat the cause not the symptoms.

In 1997, I started my website, Mercola.com, in order to educate others about taking back their health with natural medicine. Little did I know that Mercola.com would become the most visited natural health site in the world. The only problem is that the site has grown to over 100,000 pages of content and it becomes somewhat daunting to know where to start with all the information. So I chose to write this book so that you could get the best of that information into one simple program for you to follow.

Useful Principles That Work For Nearly Every Health Problem

One of the major principles I want you to understand is that your body has an enormous capacity for self-healing. It is designed to be healthy and will move in that direction once you provide it with all the essential building blocks.

I've had many patients over the years whose doctors gave them frightening disease labels and told them there wasn't anything they could do to help them (except prescribe more drugs). When these patients followed a healthy lifestyle program, they typically experienced enormous improvement. They rapidly became aware of the truth that it's about removing the obstacles to allow your body to heal itself. Remember that your body wants to move towards health and away from disease as long as you provide the environment for it to do so.

You Can Do This Program in the Comfort of Your Own Home

I have seen many thousands of patients in my clinic (The Optimal Wellness Center) improve just as dramatically as Lucy did. (See page 9)

For those with serious and complex illnesses, it would certainly make sense to seek medical advice from a qualified natural health practitioner; however, even with those that are severely ill, it is possible to get well just by following the principles I am going to share in this book.

TAKE CONTROL

Lucy And Her Battle With Kogan's Syndrome

I had a patient named Lucy with a very rare condition called Kogan's Syndrome. This syndrome is an autoimmune complication of a rheumatoid arthritis variant that causes blindness, hearing loss, and crippling arthritis in most that are afflicted.

There are only a handful of patients in the world with this condition. Lucy had been all over the world in search of an answer to her condition, consulting some of the top experts in the world, but the only hope they could offer her was to put her on dangerous and toxic anticancer medications and steroids.

When I first met Lucy, I explained the principles I reviewed above and told her that it did not matter what her symptoms were or what label she had been given, she could get better if she followed the basic program I outline in this book.

She reluctantly agreed to follow the program, although she was skeptical as no one else had offered her any ray of hope. Sure enough, just as I predicted, she started to improve and get her health back. She had a few challenges along the road, but for the most part her pain, fatigue, and disability were radically improved when she followed the program.

It is interesting to note that she is not on any "magic pills"—only some simple foundational food supplements like omega-3 fats and good bacteria.

Lucy is now featured in our newsletter each week with her videos on healthy cooking and nutrition. She is delighted to be able to inspire others to improve their health as she has done. ঌ

Believe me, I am not holding anything back. I am sharing all the "secrets" that I have learned in my 25 years of clinical practice. If you simply follow them, the overwhelming odds are that you will improve your health, and for most of you, your health will improve quite dramatically.

You will save yourself the pain and inconvenience of being crippled with a chronic illness as you age. You will look and feel young for years to come.

What Real Health is All About

"Dr. Mercola is among the few with the credentials, brains, and guts to stand up to these drug companies and remind us—with sound research and grounded commentary—what real health is all about and how to achieve it. I believe the best investment someone can make in themselves and in those they love is to learn about real health and to support this new group at the same time by buying Dr. Mercola's Take Control of Your Health program—then to read it and pass it on. Encourage others to do the same. We won't take back our health until we stop those who are keeping us from freely choosing nature over drugs."

—*Steve McCardell, Rochester, MI* ৶

You Don't Have to Spend Loads of Money on Expensive Supplements

At my clinic, the Optimal Wellness Center, we routinely see patients who bring in a literal shopping bag full of supplements. They wonder why those hundreds of dollars of supplements haven't cured them yet. We teach them that lifestyle has a much greater impact on their health than supplements and when we help them make those foundational changes, they get better.

What You Should Get Out Of Reading This Book

It is my intention to summarize the best principles I have learned in my nearly three decades of practicing medicine and in over ten years of searching the medical literature for foundational truths.

Every week I review about 5000 articles, so over the last ten years there are many hundreds of thousands of articles that have been scanned to support the health advice I provide on Mercola.com and in this book. Most of you simply would not have the time in your life to do this type of research. And why would you want to if someone like myself already does it for you for free?

After all, life is short, and there are far better things to do than research. You can benefit from this research by employing the principles set out in this book—not only will you extend the quantity of years you live but also the quality. Most people, as they get older, needlessly suffer from the pain and disability of chronic disease that sucks the joy out of their lives. If you can apply the principles in this book, you can avoid this grim fate and live a life of robust health and immense joy.

I want to be sensitive to the fact that the dietary and lifestyle changes I am encouraging you to make in this book are pretty radical. Please don't put this book down and tell yourself "I can't do this," because that would be a lie. **The truth is that you can do this.**

Thousands of people just like you have been exactly where you are at, and they have done it. Once you experience how great it is to look and feel your best, you will want to stay on track. Success breeds success and I promise you that you can be successful at becoming independently healthy, and you owe it to yourself to try. The changes may seem overwhelming to you at first. I want you to spend some time thinking about what you believe your greatest obstacle will be— then take time to make a plan.

Ask yourself "What will I do to make progress today in this area?"

For example, let's say you haven't exercised since the power went out in your office building two years ago, when you were forced to climb those eight flights of stairs to your desk. Gasping for air, you reached the 8th floor, and you promised yourself you'd start exercising—but haven't done it since.

Today is the day. A new pair of good quality shoes can be an effective motivation to start exercising. Write down "buy new shoes" on a day this week. Then schedule that 30–minute walk, and get it done. You'll feel so good.

If one of your obstacles has to do with how expensive organic food is, and you are telling yourself that you can't afford it, I am telling you that you are worth every penny spent. Additionally, you will be able to afford it more easily by eliminating the purchase of additional unhealthy foods that are making you sick. What you save on convenience foods you will more than pay back later in disease, lack of energy, time at the doctor's office or hospital and an early trip to the grave.

Stop and think about every single item you place in your grocery cart. Ask yourself "Is this good for me, or for my family?" If the answer is no then leave it on the shelf. Replace it with something you can feel good about feeding yourself, and those you love. Your cart should be very full after you leave the produce section.

Will You Have Setbacks?

Let's face it, we all have bad days. Sometimes they last for weeks. It's not an excuse to throw in the towel and just give up on your journey. The changes I am encouraging you to make are going to happen over time.

None of us are perfect.

When you have a bad day, you are probably going to feel lousy in more ways than one. Pay attention to that feeling. Journal about it— learn from it. It's not how your body was created to feel. Choose to get back on track, and make a plan to move forward. Reflect on what may have led to the setback. Often these things are completely out of our control.

Maybe you've had an exceptionally rotten day at the office, or your children have been bickering since they rolled out of bed. You don't have the energy left to prepare that healthy meal that sounded so good several days ago when you wrote it down. Give yourself grace.

Tomorrow is a new day.

You will do well to come up with a Plan B. These days will happen again, they are inevitable. Learn how you will face them the next day around.

Always remember that you can Take Control of Your Health.

Discover the Powerful Health-Building Value of Nutritional Typing & Eating Right for Your Nutritional Type

Many may not realize that I was not raised in a home that taught me any nutritional basics. I love my mother dearly, but she never had any education on how to be healthy. My mother never graduated high school and worked nights, weekends and most holidays as a waitress. My siblings and I frequently relied on highly processed foods for our meals.

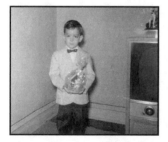

My sugar addiction begins at an early age with an Easter basket full of candy

There were plenty of snacks at my house, and I had my fair share of cookies, Pop Tarts and Hostess Twinkies. Breakfast usually consisted of cereal and perhaps white bread toast loaded with margarine, sugar and cinnamon. I continued the toast and margarine practice into my early medical school days, but I did substitute whole wheat bread for the white bread—and believed I was doing well.

Except for fruit, I rarely ate raw food. I was told that raw food could make you ill. I clearly remember one of my friends in college eating a raw pepper, and I was aghast and warned him that eating raw vegetables might make him sick! My wise friend assured me this was a healthy practice and encouraged me to consider it.

This was about the time I began to explore the importance of nutrition with a subscription to *Prevention* magazine and a series of books written by nutrition pioneer Adelle Davis.

Later I studied Nathan Pritikin, who convinced me of the importance of a diet that was high in carbohydrates and fiber and low in fat and protein. Later, I became further confused by reading and trying the *Fit For Life* diet in the late '80s.

Unfortunately, as a Protein Type (I'll explain what this is later) neither diet was designed for my Nutritional Type. Instead, they worsened my health. The "fruit only" breakfast that *Fit For Life* advocates, quickly increased my triglycerides to over 1000 so I stopped that one relatively quickly.

In my attempts to be healthy, I ate the low-fat, low-protein, high-carb diet Pritikin recommended. This was great for a Carb Type but a disaster for a Protein Type. For 20 years my diet consisted of mostly vegetarian meals such as uncooked oats with water (I thought this was healthier than cooked oatmeal), plenty of whole wheat bread, white rice, tubs of margarine, beans and produce.

This approach, combined with my running of up to 50 miles or more per week, plummeted my total cholesterol level to 75, and this was without any drugs like Lipitor. Now at that time most physicians, including myself, felt the lower your cholesterol the better. Of course, this was not correct and was actually causing health problems for me, as an optimal total cholesterol level is around 175 to 200.

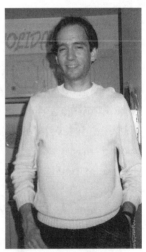

Most of my life I was thin, wiry and weak. Now at age 52, I feel like I'm in my prime. I've reached optimal health at last!

One of the primary problems with low cholesterol levels is that your body requires cholesterol as a building block to build the vast majority of your hormones. It is a foundational precursor to nearly all of your steroid hormones, and when it is low your hormones will become unbalanced.

Even though many often told me I looked gaunt and too thin, I tried to evangelize my fellow med students, patients, and anyone who would listen to eat this same way.

In medical school we had a system where the 100 students in our class would rotate and take very comprehensive notes so we would only have to take notes a few times a quarter, yet we would have everyone's comprehensive notes. This helped us study and pass our exams.

When it was my turn to take notes, no matter what the topic was, I would find a way to insert nutritional advice into the student notes. This earned me the nickname "Dr. Fiber" for my recommendation of high fiber, high-grain diets.

During my three years of family practice residency I frequently gave free nutrition lectures, but the interest was minimal. However, my enthusiasm for the high-carb, low-fat diet came to a screeching halt one fateful night when I attended a lecture by Dr. Ron Rosedale in Chicago in the fall of 1995. Dr. Rosedale opened up my eyes to how high-carb diets had the potential to increase insulin to abnormally high levels. Furthermore, he taught that keeping insulin levels in the normal range was central to optimal health and keeping disease at bay.

Eat Right for Your Blood Type Caused Me to Have Diabetes

After I understood insulin, I took another side track with Dr. Peter D'Adamo's *Eat Right for Your Blood Type* book, which appealed to me because it preached the individualization of diet based on one's blood type. There are four basic blood types, O, A, B & AB, and so four different diets are offered. Dr. D'Adamo's dietary recommendations can help to some extent—primarily because he encourages his readers to stay away from refined and processed foods and to eat whole, fresh organic foods instead.

Additionally, the most common blood type is O, and in this system blood type O's are instructed to avoid wheat and minimize consumption of almost all other grain products.

My experience has taught me that most people do tend to improve once they make these changes, so it is my impression that these were the primary reasons why some people had some success with the Blood Type Diet. Unfortunately, my blood type is A and that diet is high in grains and low in meat. This is the exact opposite of what a Protein Type like me should be eating to stay healthy. While trying this approach to diet, my fasting blood sugar rose to over 126. This means I actually developed type 2 diabetes from following this program.

This is not unusual considering 75 million people in the United States alone have diabetes and pre-diabetes, and nearly all of my paternal relatives have diabetes or have died from diabetic complications. I immediately got the clue and stopped D'Adamo's Blood Type A Diet. Although I am grateful to him for bringing attention to the concept of diet individualization, I have reached the conclusion that there is a far more important factor than just your general blood type that can help you determine what foods are best for you.

And that factor is: your metabolism. Your blood type has absolutely NO direct influence on your metabolism of protein, carbs and fats for energy. And energy metabolism is the key issue of health.

Once I started recommending that my patients decrease the amount of carbs in their diets I noticed that most of them experienced dramatic improvements in their insulin levels and overall health. I was so impressed with these results that I wrote a book about my experience called *The No Grain Diet*, which became a *New York Times* bestselling book.

However, there were still a fair number of people who did not get better with the diet that I told all my patients to follow—despite their strict compliance. I couldn't understand why.

My Experience With Vegetable Juicing

Right around the time of my experimentation with the blood type diet, I was very impressed with how healthy a few of my older patients were. There was one 70-year-old woman who had followed nutritional principles for many years, and she looked like she was 40. She believed it was due to her vegetable juicing program. So I started to research this and was impressed with the benefits of raw food vegetable juicing. I started doing it myself and recommending it to many of my patients.

Unfortunately, I had never really struggled with any serious health issues and have, for the most part, felt full of energy my entire life. So I was unable to appreciate any side effects from juicing other than I started to become allergic to some of the vegetables I was juicing on a regular basis, like Swiss chard and collard greens.

It wasn't until I learned Metabolic Typing that I would understand that the juicing would move my biochemistry in the exact opposite way I needed it to go. It was far too high in potassium for my needs and actually speeded up my already far too fast oxidation rate.

However, this type of vegetable juicing was beyond phenomenal for many of the patients I recommended it to and they had enormous benefits. Later I realized those who benefitted were the Carb Types. But my experience with many patients not improving with juicing made me far more open to the Metabolic Typing principles that I would learn in a few years.

The juicing program I developed back then is still used in our clinic and is one of the more popular pages on my Web site. Mercola.com has ranked number one or two for the term "vegetable juicing" on Google for the past five years. We still strongly recommend that all of our Carb Type patients adopt this juicing plan to achieve a high level of health.

The positive benefits many of my patients experienced with vegetable juicing helped convince me of the importance of raw food and really set the stage for my future experimentation with raw animal foods.

My Next Nutritional Health Epiphany—Metabolic Typing™

Dr. Rosedale's insights on insulin were finally some of the nutritional golden truths that I had been searching for, for so many years. Nothing I have learned since then has altered or changed my views of these truths. In fact, it has been quite the contrary. Most people have experienced profound improvements in their health, once their insulin levels have normalized.

The next stop on my nutritional journey occurred in early 2001 when I finally understood the reason that a significant number of people did not respond to the insulin-control program I had developed. That is when I encountered Bill Wolcott's book *The Metabolic Typing Diet*, which carefully explained that there are three basic types of human metabolism:

- Carb Type metabolism

- Protein Type metabolism

- Mixed Type metabolism

People metabolize the food they eat in different ways based mostly on their genetics, but a number of other factors, such as chronic stress, can also influence our metabolic activity. According to Metabolic Typing, people can be classified as either Carb Types, Protein Types or Mixed Types, based on how they answer a computerized questionnaire. Also, there are two different kinds of Carb Types, two different kinds of Protein Types and two different kinds of Mixed Types.

Discovering Metabolic Typing was a major epiphany for me and explained the years of frustration I was having in trying to fit everyone into the same nutritional model.

There Is No Perfect Diet For Everyone

Once I adopted Metabolic Typing into my practice, the patients who previously had not responded well to our program started to improve. I will be eternally grateful to Bill Wolcott for revolutionizing the way I practiced medicine. It is my belief that Metabolic Typing and understanding the importance of insulin control are the two most important principles of successful nutrition counseling; they are both deserving of the nutritional equivalent of the Nobel Prize.

I had previously recommended fresh organic vegetable juice to everyone, but realized after learning about Metabolic Typing that this has the greatest value for Carb Types. It has less value for most Mixed Types and the least value for Protein Types.

Metabolic Typing helped me to finally understand that the high-protein, low-carb diet I had been advocating as a starting point to all of my patients to normalize insulin levels, was a disaster for Carb Types. These people actually needed a dietary approach higher in healthy forms of carbohydrates.

Now, it is important to understand that I didn't abandon all of the nutritional principles I had acquired prior to learning about Metabolic Typing, such as eating lots of fresh, raw, organic whole foods. My team and I actually incorporated this strong emphasis on food quality at the very beginning of our practice of Metabolic Type nutrition.

We also made the discovery—after just a few months of practicing Metabolic Type nutrition—that it is not enough to make the right food choices, it is equally important to eat your foods—at each meal—in the right order!

For instance, which food do you think would be the best one for Protein Types to eat first at any given meal—<u>meat</u> or a vegetable? Which food do you think would be the best one for Carb Types to eat first at any given meal—meat or a <u>vegetable</u>? And, which food do you think would be the best one for Mixed Types to eat first at any given meal—meat or a vegetable?

Protein Types should eat their meat first, Carb Types should eat their vegetable first and Mixed Types should eat their meat and vegetable together! When this is faithfully practiced, digestive and meta-bolic efficiency typically improves dramatically. This is indicated by:

- Improved meal satisfaction (and with smaller portions of food)
- No need for snacks in between meals
- No more food cravings

Over the course of the five years that we have been using Metabolic Typing, we have identified what is most valuable about the system. We started with, and eliminated, what we have learned is unnecessary and burdensome. We've made big nutritional improvements that have helped our patients to often experience dramatic and even amazing improvements in their health within the first month of eating right for their Nutritional Type.

When I told other clinicians who were doing Metabolic Typing with their patients how we had improved the Metabolic Type nutrition plans, I was surprised to hear that they were all eager to learn about what we were doing. This was because many of them had actually stopped using Metabolic Typing in their practice because it was simply too complex and burdensome for the average patient to successfully implement.

Our experience with thousands of patients has confirmed for us, over and over again, that we have identified the most important nutritional principles that help people to achieve dramatically improved health, without burdensome effort.

Raw Food Exploration

After I had become comfortable with Metabolic Typing, I learned more about the Weston Price Foundation with Sally Fallon and Mary Enig. Their compelling literature started my raw food exploration by using raw dairy. It took nearly two years to locate an Amish farmer in Michigan who could drive dairy to my Chicago-area clinic, but it was well worth the wait. I observed yet another improvement boost among many of our patients who were able to access raw, unpasteurized dairy.

From there I progressed to one of the only teachers of **raw animal foods**, Aajonus Vanderplanitz. Vanderplanitz teaches that humans are the only species that cooks their meat. All other animals eat their food and meat raw. Vanderplanitz was able to recover from some very serious medical problems by eating a raw food diet and he has helped many people do the same.

While I don't agree with everything that Vanderplanitz teaches, especially his liberal use of raw honey, he has uncovered many helpful principles and his work is part of our new system called Nutritional Typing.

Distinctions Between Metabolic Typing (MT) and Nutritional Typing (NT)

Simplified Categorization

MT categorizes people into three main metabolic types, but there are six subtypes and nine possible Metabolic Typing combinations. In our experience, all you really need to know is: Are you a Protein Type, Carb Type or Mixed Type?

Food Quality

One of the most important distinctions between these two systems has to do with attention to food quality. For example, MT emphasizes specific foods to eat but does not strongly emphasize the quality of these foods. On the other hand, NT advocates that buying the highest quality food that is available to you is vital. Not only do we advise and help our patients obtain fresh, locally grown, organic food, but we also recommend that you eat as much of your food raw as possible. Eating raw will serve to preserve the nutritional integrity of your food.

If you do cook your food, and we know that most people will, then it is very important to use our low-temperature cooking guidelines as often as possible, as this will minimize the amount of heat damage that you cause to your food.

You might already be familiar with the differences between raw and pasteurized milk. Well, similarly, if you cook (i.e. heat damage) other foods, they will lose much of their ability to transfer their vital nutrients to your body.

Supplementation

MT advocates that everyone should take a number of supplements (multi-vitamins, enzymes and other products) designed for their type.

However, NT does not at all focus on nutritional supplementation as a primary means of improving your health. The primary approach is to use food and rely on supplements only when indicated for specialized conditions. It has been our experience that taking supplements hardly ever helps people make big, nor lasting, improvements in their health.

Overall Nutritional Differences

MT nutrition plans emphasize making the right food choices based not only on whether you're a Protein, Carb or Mixed Type, but also takes into account your endocrine type and, yes, even your blood type (although the list of blood-type-related foods to avoid are much shorter and different than what Dr. D'Adamo teaches).

MT also emphasizes that you should be focused on the percentages and ratios of protein, carbs and fat that you are eating at each meal. (It's not surprising that many of our patients became confused when we were practicing this approach.)

In NT, the emphasis is on making the right food choices for your basic type—Protein, Carb or Mixed—together with a big emphasis on food quality and eating foods raw. Plus, emphasis is placed on the best ways to cook your food, IF you are going to cook it, and always consuming your most metabolically important food or foods FIRST, thereby practicing the right kind of food combining for your Nutritional Type. Last but not least, eating consciously is an incredibly important facet of NT!

This is all much easier to do and, we feel, far more effective at improving your digestive and metabolic efficiency than focusing on making food choices based on three different, and sometimes contradictory, concerns (Metabolic Type, endocrine type and blood type), along with focusing on the percentages and ratios of protein, carbs and fat that you are eating at each meal while taking lots of supplements.

Also, we strongly prefer the term "Nutritional Typing," over "Metabolic Typing" because the emphasis is on NUTRITION. And, ultimately Nutritional or Metabolic Typing is only a means to an end, which is: knowing how to truly nourish yourself in the way that you truly need to be nourished.

I have collaborated with about half a dozen leading nutrition experts who were trained in Metabolic Typing, who felt that the system needed to be revised and simplified. We have developed our own system for determining whether you are a Protein, Carb or Mixed type and this revolutionary and cutting-edge refinement was developed in the spring of 2007. It is literally hot off the press. This information does not exist in written form ANYWHERE else in the world. It is my belief that helping develop and provide an easy system for individualizing your ideal diet may be the single most important contribution I ever make.

The potential for this program to improve your health is beyond extraordinary. It has been our observation that most of the people who faithfully apply NT observe phenomenal improvements in their health.

Why Do You Need Nutritional Typing?

Your Nutritional Type determines your individual nutritional requirements and dictates your individual responses to what you eat and drink. Foods and individual nutrients do not behave the same way in people with different Nutritional Types.

So what exactly is your Nutritional Type?

Your nutritional type is primarily determined by your genetically inherited ability to metabolize various foods into the energy and building blocks your body needs to be healthy. However, environmental influences, such as stress, can cause a functional adaptation in your metabolism that temporarily overrides your genetics. Ultimately, your Nutritional Type, at any given time in your life, is determined by identifying the primary characteristics of your metabolism.

And identifying your basic Nutritional Type is really quite simple because there are only three basic types: Protein Types, Carb Types and Mixed Types. While there can be significant variations within each one of these three basic types, everyone on this planet, at any given time, will have a Protein, Carb or Mixed Type metabolism.

Why Nutritional Typing is NOT Just Another Fad Diet

Tens of thousands of books have been written on dieting and nutrition in the past 100 years, each one with its own principles and teachings. Sometimes the diets seem to work, other times not, and often they help one person but are devastating to another. For example, some people feel great on the Atkins Diet (low-carb) and quickly lose excess weight. Meanwhile, other people have reported feeling sick, tired, moody and have **gained weight** on a low-carb diet.

Unfortunately, nearly all of the dietary recommendations that you read or hear promote a single regimen or approach as being ideal or appropriate for everyone who applies it. Remember that I have made this mistake too—several times.

And this is a terrible mistake in that it completely fails to appreciate the proven fact that we do not all have the same nutritional requirements. Certain foods or a diet that works well for one person may actually cause health problems for someone else. Unfortunately, this profound truth is not "officially" acknowledged by the vast majority of doctors, dieticians, nutritionists and other health care practitioners, and it took me years to learn this for myself.

We have all been subjected to general and often vague food recommendations by so-called experts, even though it has been over 2,000 years since the ancient Roman philosopher Lucretius observed the profound truth that "What is food to one man may be fierce poison to others." (Over the years, this statement was re-phrased, and in modern times it is most commonly known as "One man's food is another man's poison.")

Just as you are unique in regard to your outward physical characteristics, you also are unique with respect to your inner biochemistry and physiology. There is actually a spectrum of possible variations that exist in the way people digest and metabolize foods.

When it comes to digestion and metabolism, however, there is much that you also have in common with others. For instance, we all need to be able to digest and metabolize protein. What makes NT so different from any other "diet" you may have tried is that it guides you to the foods that are the right sources of protein for you, together with teaching you how to optimize the metabolic value of the protein.

Remember, what's right for you could be very wrong for someone else, because although we all have much in common with each other, we do have our differences—and it's our differences that make us unique.

The Details ARE Important

Granted, our differences are mostly in the details, but never underestimate the importance of details. You may not have thought much about the nutritional differences between the white meat and dark meat of poultry, but in Nutritional Typing it is known that there is a significant difference in the value of these two foods.

Also consider the molecular formula for hemoglobin (which is the part of a red blood cell that picks up and carries oxygen) is $C_{738}H_{1166}FeN_{203}O_{208}S_2$ (C=Carbon, H=Hydrogen, Fe=Iron, N=Nitrogen, O=Oxygen & S=Sulfur). Hemoglobin is a molecule containing 2,318 atoms, and only one of those atoms is iron. Compared to the entire structure of hemoglobin, the one atom of iron could be viewed as a very minor detail. But that one very minor detail makes it possible for the cells of your body to receive the oxygen that they need, without which, you would die.

So the lesson here is: *never take the details for granted!*

Nutritional Typing gives more attention to the specific details of what you are eating than any other school of nutrition, diet book or fad diet in history! And you will want to give faithful attention to the details that we teach you once you experience the benefits of doing so.

It is Highly Likely You Have Never Experienced Optimal Health

It may sound shocking, but it's absolutely true. It's likely that you haven't yet experienced optimum health. What does optimum health feel like? It's:

- Having more energy than you know what to do with

- Being free from aches and pains

- Feeling happy, optimistic and at peace emotionally

Being optimally healthy means that you feel this way almost always, as opposed to feeling this way only rarely when you're having a "good day."

It is not your fault, though, that you likely haven't reached this level of health. Our culture is intertwined with pervasive corporate interests that are directly aligned with their self-serving profit motives. It is designed to make these companies successful, often at the expense of people's long-term health.

NT Shows You How to Use Food as Your Medicine

Part of what our culture promotes is a medical system based on treating symptoms, and not addressing the underlying cause of those symptoms. Because of this, conventional medicine, although highly effective for many acute health challenges, really has a very limited ability to resolve most all chronic illnesses. Therapeutically, this approach or paradigm is known as allopathic medicine.

If you want a powerful visual analogy of this concept please view the seven-minute animation I created a few years ago that demonstrates this. You can see it at:

Mercola.com/Allopath

Unfortunately, much of contemporary alternative medicine falls under the same strategic approach. This stems from the lack of technology to effectively analyze and resolve the biochemical imbalances that are the underlying cause of disease.

This is not so with NT, however. Nutritional Typing is unlike conventional medicine and most alternative medicine modalities in its unique ability to:

- Balance your total body chemistry

- Address disease processes at their causative level

- Prevent illness

- Rebuild health

- Provide uniquely long-lasting health benefits

When you begin eating right for your Nutritional Type, you will also begin to move toward metabolic balance. And as you move toward metabolic balance your body will be producing energy more efficiently from the foods that you're eating.

When you are in metabolic balance, you will then discover what it feels like to be truly healthy. You will have created an inner environment that is conducive to you experiencing your highest levels of:

- Peaceful energy

- Relaxed alertness

- Emotional poise

- Positive stable mood

- Great mental clarity

NT works for those who are healthy and those who are experiencing health challenges. If your body is in need of healing, you will be helping yourself realize your full healing potential. If you feel that you are already healthy, you're in for a surprise! You will create the possibility of truly knowing just how healthy you can be.

How Will I Know I'm Eating Right for My Nutritional Type?

You will experience a profound difference in the way you feel before and after you begin eating right for your Nutritional Type. When you are NOT eating right for your Nutritional Type you typically:

- Do not feel satisfied with your meals

- Have cravings, especially for sugar

- Have frequent and intense hunger (especially true for Protein Types)

- Experience mood swings

- Experience some degree of 'brain fog'
- Have inconsistent and/or low energy
- Are more prone to feeling anxious and depressed
- Are more prone to addictions
- Will be very prone to being overweight or underweight
- Are prone to all types of degenerative processes

Meanwhile, at the other end of the spectrum, when you ARE eating right for your Nutritional Type you typically:

- Will be more satisfied with your meals
- Can go for longer periods without eating
- Are completely FREE from ALL cravings
- Experience a more positive and stable mood
- Experience elimination of 'brain fog' and heightened levels of mental clarity
- Experience more consistently good energy
- Lose weight if you are overweight and gain weight if you are underweight
- Support on-going cellular repair and regeneration
- Begin to realize your full health potential

The Principles of Nutritional Typing

There are five primary principles that you will need to focus on to successfully eat right for your Nutritional Type. The first three principles are actually of equal importance, but we will list them here in the order that they will need to be addressed as you shop and then plan and prepare your meals:

1. Make the right food choices. Initially, choose all of your foods from your Nutritional Type food chart. Buy the best quality food that is available to you.

2. Consider what you will eat RAW and what you will eat COOKED. When cooking, *never* overcook your food. Use low-temperature cooking as often as you can.

3. Always consume your most metabolically important food or foods FIRST! For example, if you are a Protein Type eat your meat first, if you are a Carb Type eat your vegetables first and if you are a Mixed type eat your meat and vegetables together.

4. Practice the right kind of food combining for your Nutritional Type. (This is especially important for MIXED types.)

5. Eat consciously! Pay attention to what you are eating and—if you do not already do so—then begin to practice eating slowly and chewing your food thoroughly.

When you put these five principles into practice, you then set yourself up for success with principle number six, which has to do with those perplexing percentages and ratios of protein, carbs and fat that you are eating at each meal.

6. The truth is: the amounts of protein, fat and carbohydrates that you are eating at each meal are definitely important—**but please do not think about this in terms of percentages and ratios.** The amount of protein, fat and carbs that you eat is also known as the macronutrient ratio, and it is the most dynamic part of eating right for your Nutritional Type. But, the correct macronutrient ratio for you can vary depending on a number of factors, including your levels of stress and activity, and also the climate where you are living.

Perhaps you have heard about the macronutrient ratio, as it is the subject of a book called "The Zone Diet." This book proposes that to get in the "zone" a person should strive to eat 40 percent of their calories from carbs, 30 percent from protein and 30 percent from fat.

However, this is incredibly misleading, as there is NO macronutrient ratio that is right for everyone all the time. (It's another one-size-fits-all approach.) As indicated above, even your own ideal macronutrient ratio can vary significantly from time to time.

So how do you get your ideal amounts of protein, fat and carbs right at every meal without turning your meal into a complex mathematical problem?

The answer is simple: Focus on making the right food choices (principle #1) and eating your food in the right way (principles 2, 3, 4 & 5). As for how much you should eat of any given food in your meal plan, initially, you should let your appetite be your guide, then learn from your experience.

You must always listen carefully to your body, trust what it tells you and remember what you have learned.

If you pay attention, your own body language (how you feel physically, mentally and emotionally) will always let you know if you are or are not nourishing yourself correctly. So while the macronutrient ratio is important, so is figuring out your best macronutrient ratio in an intuitive way, rather than in an intellectual way!

There is one more principle that needs to be addressed, especially for those of you who do take nutritional supplements. And that brings us to principle number seven, which is:

7. Only take supplements that are right for your Nutritional Type. Avoid supplements that are wrong for your Nutritional Type.

While the right supplements for your Nutritional Type can definitely be helpful, they are not essential for most people to experience dramatic and even amazing health improvements. If you are on a tight budget, always prioritize spending your money on the best-quality food that is right for your Nutritional Type rather than spending it on supplements.

Raw Foods and Low-Temperature Cooking

The second NT principle is all about how you prepare your foods, so ideally you will want to eat them either raw or lightly cooked. Consuming foods in this form ensures that you get the maximum nutritional value from the foods, and the least amount of toxic byproducts.

You may not realize that cooking foods, particularly at high temperatures, actually creates health-harming compounds in the food, and this is something you definitely want to avoid. Eating foods as close to their natural form as possible is a primary goal with NT.

So, whenever possible you should seek out organic raw foods. This includes raw organic fruits and vegetables, organic raw dairy products like raw milk, raw kefir, and raw yogurt, and organic raw meats and seafood like steak tartar and salmon tartar, all according to your NT, of course.

However, raw dairy products can be very difficult to come by in the United States. If you cannot find a source of raw dairy products, you can substitute organic pasteurized dairy products, if they are agreeable to your body. Meanwhile, some people are opposed to eating raw meats and seafood. For this reason, it's acceptable to lightly cook your foods using low-temperature cooking.

Low-temperature cooking conserves more of the naturally occurring moisture and flavor in the food, plus, the food does not stick to the cookware. Most importantly, the food will be easier for your body to properly digest, and you will be conserving much more of the nutritional value of the food.

Low-Temperature Cooking Guidelines:

- Use a glass casserole dish with a cover. (The cover is very important.) The tighter the cover fits, the better. The size of the casserole dish should be appropriate for the amount of food being cooked. In other words, the casserole dish should be about the same size as what you are cooking, and should not be too big.

- Cook your food in the oven at 225 degrees Fahrenheit—*No Higher!*

- Allow for 12 to15 minutes of cooking time per each 4 ounces of food being cooked, but decrease or increase the cooking time as needed.

Other healthy methods of cooking that are acceptable to use with NT include crock-pot cooking, poaching, steaming your food lightly or searing your food (on the outside, and leaving the inside very rare).

The Essential NT Guidelines: Protein Types

Protein Types can eat high-quality sources of protein and fat very freely, but they need to be very careful with their carbohydrate intake. It is very easy for a Protein Type to over-consume carbohydrates!

Contrary to the name, though, just because you are a Protein Type does not mean you need large amounts of protein. You may, in fact, need as little as 1 or 2 ounces of protein per meal depending on a variety of factors, including how much you weigh. But as little as one ounce of the right kind of protein could be enough to satisfy your body's need for protein—as long as you *eat it first and finish it completely* before you eat any other food.

Here are some tendencies and characteristics of Protein Types:

- They have strong appetites
- They tend to think about food a lot, even when they're not hungry
- They do not do well with fasting
- They do not feel well (especially mood wise) if they skip a meal
- When they crave sugar or refined carbs, it will feel good to them in the moment if they eat some (but eating sugar or refined carbs will never satisfy a Protein Type's cravings for long)
- Eating sugar or refined carbs will typically stimulate their desire for more sugar or refined carbs
- They also have cravings for fatty, salty foods, and these foods have a more satisfying effect
- They will feel hungry most of the time if they eat a low-fat or vegetarian-type diet

TAKE CONTROL	**No More Food Cravings, Plus Weight Loss!**

No More Food Cravings, Plus Weight Loss!

Shirley is 63 years young and is a retired nurse. She has a long history of being overweight and having heart palpitations. As a new patient, she was about 100 pounds overweight and had failed on all of the diet programs she tried. She was simply unable to sustain any significant weight loss.

Shirley started having heart palpitations in 1988 while getting ready for her daughter's graduation. Eventually, she was given the effective but dangerous calcium channel blocker Verapamil, which she continues to take—although, she reports that she has not had heart palpitations for about 10 years.

In Nutritional Typing, she was assessed as a Protein Type. Her comprehensive blood test clearly indicated that she had been over-consuming carbohydrates, (Her insulin level was 10 and her leptin level was 29.4. Also, she was deficient in vitamin D (18)).

For three months, Shirley followed the prime Protein Type meal plan as faithfully as she could and she continues to feel much better. Specifically, her mood has dramatically improved, her energy is about 80 percent better, her mental clarity is sharper and it continues to improve.

The most remarkable aspect, though, is that she continues to be completely free of cravings for carbohydrates. After a meal she can easily go for about six hours before she feels a need to eat again. Additionally, after some adjustments were made in her portions of protein, fat and carbohydrates at every meal, she has lost 11 pounds—without dieting.

—*Shirley D, East Windsor, New Jersey* ᔒ

The Prime Protein Type Meal Plan Guidelines

Protein type foods typically have the following characteristics:

- Higher in total fat

- Lower in total carbohydrate

- Vegetables carbohydrates are relatively low in potassium and most green leafy vegetables are avoided

- Protein sources are high in purine amino acids, so dark red meats like beef, lamb, and dark poultry are preferable

The table for protein type foods is not easily displayed in this book format so it is freely available at my web site: You will also find a link on that page that allows you to take the computerized nutritional typing test that can help you identify which nutritional type you are.

Mercola.com/ProteinType

Protein Types should follow the following guidelines with their meal plans for optimal health:

1. Choose ALL of your foods from the Protein Type food chart following these guidelines (except any foods that you are allergic, intolerant or sensitive to).

2. Give faithful attention to food quality, eating fresh, organic food as often as possible and, ideally, only eating meats from healthy, humanely raised animals.

3. Follow our three-part Protein Type meal plan for your breakfast, lunch and dinner. Each meal should be eaten in three separate parts (think in terms of a three-course meal). Parts one and two are ESSENTIAL, but part three is optional:

Part 1: Eat high-quality meat, fowl, fish or seafood listed on the Protein Type food chart at EVERY meal, and ALWAYS eat a serving of meat, fowl, fish or seafood **first. Finish it completely** before you touch any carbohydrates!

Remember, as little as 1 or 2 ounces of meat, fowl, fish or seafood may be enough for you at any meal. However, feel free to eat the amount of meat, fowl, fish or seafood that feels right to you.

Part 2: Consume some very low-carb and/or low-carb vegetable nutrition with every meal. Also, consume at least one of the following complementary *foods along* with your vegetable nutrition:

Raw Cream	Olives	Seeds
Raw Butter	Olive Oil	Nuts
Raw Cheese	Coconut	Nut Butters
Raw Cottage Cheese	Coconut Cream	
Avocado	Coconut Oil	

Part 3: You may consume any of the following *in small amounts*, and only at the *very end of your meal* or not at all:

Artichoke Hearts	White Potato	Apple
Carrots	Winter Squash	Pear
Peas	Chestnuts	Banana
Beans	Raw Milk	Cranberries
Lentils	Raw Kefir	
Whole Grains	Raw Yogurt	

Do not eat any of these foods at the start of a meal or in between meals. Also, when eating Part 3 foods, always eat them with some additional high-quality fat or oil.

4. Focus on making the right food choices and eating in the right way. This means always eat your most metabolically important food first (Part 1) and eat the other foods at your meal in the right order (Parts 2 and 3). As for how much you should eat, initially let your appetite be your guide and learn from your experience. Listen to your body and trust what it tells you.

5. Eat consciously. Pay attention to what you are eating and if you do not already do so, then begin to practice eating slowly and chewing your food thoroughly.

6. If you need a snack in between meals, choose any of the foods from the Protein Type food chart that are printed in black. The foods from the chart that are printed in red should NEVER be eaten as snacks in between meals.

7. To help yourself fall asleep and stay asleep, feel free to eat a Protein-Type-appropriate snack before going to bed (but be careful to not overeat).

TAKE CONTROL	**Extreme Anxiety Relief (Protein Type)**

Extreme Anxiety Relief (Protein Type)

Jon is a 44-year-old, highly successful entrepreneur who was running a half-billion-dollar company. He was referred to me by a close friend for an 11-year history of chronic anxiety that had failed to respond to some of the best psychotherapy in the country, including EFT.

Please understand that this anxiety was nearly debilitating and crippled him from leading a normal life. It was an enormous hardship for him to run his business with this type of handicap.

What made the issue even more interesting is that he had a phenomenally healthy lifestyle. Aside from being successful in business he had also competed as a semi-professional athlete and was in excellent health. He clearly did not have an exercise deficiency.

He chose healthy foods but this turned out to be his Achilles heel. Although they were healthy, biodynamic, organic foods they were not correct for his metabolic type. In fact, they were the exact opposite of what his body required.

He was essentially eating a very healthy vegetarian, low-fat diet. Once we did his Nutritional Type and found out that he was a Protein Type, miracles occurred.

His anxiety rapidly resolved by over 90 percent until he went off his program and avoided the extra fat and protein that his body required.

Jon did find that eating a small amount of grain after eating some of his high-purine meat and vegetables has worked to completely satisfy his appetite until his next meal. He still does experience a little bit of stress-related anxiety, but he no longer experiences anxiety for no particular reason.

—Jon, St. Charles, IL ≈

Optimal Meal Ideas for Protein Types

When you receive the food chart for your specific NT, you will be free to create meals using any of your recommended foods. Here we've compiled a few ideas to get you started.

- Have a rare rib eye steak or some steak tartar, finish this completely, and then have a spinach and mushroom omelet (and finish it completely). (If this seems like a lot of food, remember you can eat as little as 1 ounce of each.)Then, if desired, end this meal with some fresh apple slices slathered with raw almond butter* and topped off with walnuts. (*Mix some freshly ground flaxseed meal into the raw almond butter.)

- Have a seared flank steak, finish this completely, and then have an organic baby spinach salad with mushroom caps, avocado, olives, pistachio nuts and pumpkin seeds. Top off the salad with some chopped chives and as much olive oil as desired. Finish the salad completely and then have one or two artichoke hearts with high-lignan flaxseed oil drizzled on top.

- Have some salmon tartar or smoked salmon (lox), finish this completely, and then have a salad made with organic baby spinach leaves, asparagus tips and sliced mushroom caps (no stems) mixed with olive oil and fresh dill. Finish the salad completely and then have some Protein Type 'Banana Cream Pudding' made by blending 1 raw egg, 1 or 2 heaping tablespoons of raw cream and a small partly green banana.

- Have some sliced roast beef, finish this completely, and then have some Protein Type 'Cole Slaw' (made with freshly grated cauliflower and raw cream, seasoned with salt and pepper). Finish this completely and then have 4-6 ounces of yogurt mixed with some freshly ground flaxseed meal and chopped walnuts.

- Have one to three chicken legs (cold or hot), finish this completely, and then have some celery stalks dipped into organic peanut butter.* Finish this completely and then if desired have a small serving of oatmeal with raw cream or raw butter, plus some chopped walnuts and cinnamon sprinkled on top. (*Mix some freshly ground flaxseed meal into the organic peanut butter.)

- Have some thinly sliced strips of raw salmon fillet with a small amount of salmon roe (caviar) on top of each slice of salmon fillet (or to keep it real simple have a can of sardines), finish this completely and then have some steamed asparagus with half of an avocado. Finish this completely and then end this meal with a serving of peas and carrots along with lots of raw butter.

- Have some ground beef, bison, or dark-meat turkey, finish this completely and then have some 'mock mashed potatoes' (made with thoroughly steamed and then mashed cauliflower plus lots of raw butter). Finish the mock mashed potatoes completely, and then end this meal with Protein Type 'Coconut-Banana Cream Pudding' (made by blending 1 raw egg, 1/4 cup of raw cream, 1/4 cup of fresh coconut meat chopped into small pieces and a small partly green banana).

- Have a whole chicken leg (with the thigh), finish this completely and then have 3-4 ounces of fresh celery/spinach juice with 1-2 ounces of raw cream and 1 raw egg mixed into the juice. Finish this completely and then end this meal with some fresh organic corn on the cob along with lots of raw butter and a sprinkle of salt.

- Have some duck breast, finish this completely, and then have steamed asparagus, cauliflower and string beans with lots of raw butter. Finish this completely and end this meal with a small pear that is sliced and slathered with raw almond butter.* (*Mix some freshly ground flaxseed meal into the raw almond butter.)

The Essential NT Guidelines: Carb Types

Carb Types can eat high-quality sources of carbohydrates very freely, but they need to be careful with their intake of protein–and they need to be even more careful with their intake of fat. It is very easy for a Carb Type to over-consume fat.

So people who are Carb Types need a diet compromised of relatively small amounts of proteins and fat compared to carbs. Excess fat and protein will leave them feeling drained and sluggish or even hyper, wired, quick to anger and irritable. It's important for Carb Types to eat low-fat (*but NOT non-fat*) foods.

They generally need to avoid red meats, with the exception of ostrich, and when they eat meat it should be light-colored fish, the white meat of chicken or turkey, or all of the meat from a cornish hen, as these are low-purine proteins. Carb Types typically do well with grains, especially if they are not struggling with elevated insulin problems like extra weight, diabetes, high cholesterol or high blood pressure, but grains are NOT their primary source of carbohydrates—vegetables are!

Here are the typical characteristics of a Carb Type:

- They have relatively light appetites
- They don't think about food much, unless they are hungry
- They have a high tolerance for carbs
- They can skip a meal, if they have to, and it doesn't hurt their energy or mood
- They can enhance their feeling of well-being through fasting
- They typically don't like meat
- They typically don't like adding salt to their food
- They love salads
- They feel great after drinking fresh, organic vegetable juice
- They feel good after drinking freshly squeezed orange juice

The table for carb type foods is not easily displayed in this book format so it is freely available at my web site: You will also find a link on that page that allows you to take the computerized nutritional typing test that can help you identify which nutritional type you are.

 Diabetes Improves on HIGH-Carb Diet!

Paula is a 64-year-old diabetic and she has struggled with high triglycerides and very high cholesterol. Her comprehensive blood test clearly indicated insulin-resistant type 2 diabetes.

Her previous physician enriched the drug companies by prescribing Lipitor, a drug that in no way, shape or form treats the cause of the problem but gives Pfizer a cool $13 billion a year in revenues. Fortunately, she could not tolerate it. (She probably got a 'thank you' note from her liver for stopping the Lipitor!)

Paula is five feet tall and was about 30 pounds overweight when she visited the Optimal Wellness Center in April of 2006. As a new patient, she expressed frustration that:

"No matter what I do, I just can't seem to lose weight and keep it off."

She also reported that she loves desserts. In fact, she has a history of having strong cravings for sugar and bread. (Cravings for sugar or bread or other refined grain products are ALWAYS a big clue that someone is NOT eating right for their type of metabolism.)

Through Nutritional Typing, Paula was identified as a strong Carb Type. Well, it took Paula some time to do the planning and preparation necessary before she could consistently eat right for her NT, but, in the middle of June 2006, she did begin to follow our prime Carb Type nutrition plan about 90 percent to 95 percent of the time.

Over the course of the next four to five months, Paula realized the following benefits:

- She experienced a huge reduction in her cravings for sugar and bread

- Her Carb Type meals were so satisfying to her, she could easily go for five to six hours after breakfast and lunch before she began to feel hungry again
- Her energy, stamina, mood and mental clarity all improved
- She lost 18.25 pounds—Without Dieting!

All of these benefits really helped to improve the quality of Paula's daily life. From a blood chemistry perspective, the value of our Carb Type nutrition plan was shown in the dramatic improvements she realized from her first blood test in April, compared to her second blood test in September.

It is important to keep in mind that these improvements began to be achieved when Paula started to eat right for her NT and used food as her medicine! Also, keep in mind that she is 64 years of age and she had only been eating right for her NT for three months when her blood test was repeated.

Test results from April 28, 2006

- Insulin: 13
- Glucose: 144
- Triglycerides: 238
- Total Cholesterol: 298
- HDL's: 45
- LDL's: 205

Test results from September 21, 2006

- Insulin: 5
- Glucose: 85
- Triglycerides: 125
- Total Cholesterol: 259
- HDL's: 48
- LDL's: 186

She Did NOT Take Any Prescription Drugs!

Paula's insulin and glucose levels from September are not only no longer at diabetic levels—these levels are outstandingly healthy for a Carb Type in her age group.

Her levels of triglycerides, total cholesterol, HDL's & LDL's still have lots of room for further improvement, but she is NO longer at high risk for heart disease. In fact, every day that she eats right for her Nutritional Type she moves further away from disease and she gets closer and closer to realizing her full health potential at this time of her life.

—*Paula, Fruit Heights, Utah* ๛

Mercola.com/CarbType

The Prime Carb Type Meal Plan Guidelines

When you receive your Carb Type food chart, you will know which foods are ideal for your type of metabolism. Here are the guidelines to follow to make each meal a movement toward excellent health:

1. Make a commitment to choose all of your foods from the Carb Type food chart following these guidelines (except any foods that you are allergic, intolerant or sensitive to).

2. Eat fresh, organic food as often as possible and consider what you will eat raw and what you will eat cooked. When cooking, never overcook your food. Use low-temperature cooking as often as you can.

3. Drink three servings a day of fresh, organic vegetable juice. Each serving of juice should be between 8 and 16 ounces.

4. **Start every meal with some fresh, organic, RAW vegetable or fruit nutrition. Drinking fresh, organic vegetable juice that includes a small amount of fruit is a great way for a Carb Type to start every meal.**

5. At least two-thirds of the vegetable nutrition in each serving of juice should come from the very-low-carb and/or low-carb vegeta-

bles (you can check your Carb Type food chart for vegetable classifications).

6. If you do not have fresh, organic vegetable juice available to you then start your meal with 6 to 8 ounces of **freshly** squeezed orange juice, or simply eat some **whole and raw**, fresh, organic vegetable or fruit nutrition, such as a tomato, an orange or an apple. Or, you could have a vegetable salad with lettuce, cherry tomatoes, bell pepper and cucumber plus a small amount of fruit such as pineapple or kiwi.

7. Be sure to eat Carb-Type-appropriate proteins. Breakfast proteins include:

- Cooked egg whites with just a small amount of cooked yolk
- A whole raw egg
- Low-fat yogurt, low-fat kefir, low-fat milk or low-fat cottage cheese
- Whole grains (especially oats) may also have enough protein to satisfy a Carb Type's need for protein at breakfast

Lunch proteins include:

- Low-fat cheese, low-fat cottage cheese, low-fat yogurt, low-fat kefir, low-fat milk
- A whole raw egg
- One whole cooked egg plus two or three additional cooked egg whites
- Light-colored fish, chicken breast or turkey breast

Dinner proteins include:

- Cornish hen, chicken breast, turkey breast, light-colored fish or ostrich
- A whole raw egg
- One whole cooked egg plus two or three additional cooked egg whites

- Low-fat cheese, low-fat cottage cheese, low-fat yogurt, low-fat kefir or low-fat milk

8. Eat two salads a day, one with lunch and one with dinner.

9. If you need a snack in between meals, choose any of the vegetables or fruits from the Carb Type food chart that are printed in black. The foods that are printed in red should NOT be eaten as snacks in between meals. Low-fat dairy products may also be included with your snack foods.

10. Focus on making the right food choices and eating in the right way. This means always eat your most metabolically important foods *first*, which for Carb Types are fresh, organic, raw vegetables and/or fruits. Also, eat consciously. Pay attention to what you are eating and if you do not already do so, then begin to practice eating slowly and chewing your food thoroughly. Initially, let your appetite be your guide when deciding how much to eat. Listen to your body and trust what it tells you.

TAKE CONTROL

Blood Pressure Improves Dramatically

The story below is from someone who had struggled with very high blood pressure for some time. She had applied the Atkins-type, low-carb, high-protein diet for her blood pressure challenge and it failed miserably. She was even eating organic foods!

Why did it fail? Because she was a Carb Type. If she were a protein type she would have had phenomenal results, just like many of the successful Atkins proponents.

Fortunately, she was a subscriber to our site and had taken our online NT test that provided her with the correct diet recommendations for her and, as you can see by her story below, it worked like an absolute charm.

Mieltje is a 54-year-old woman who had her thyroid removed in1984. She gained quite a bit of weight over the years and also had high blood pressure. She had always been able to control high blood pressure with magnesium, but lately that had not worked.

Here is her story:

"After 10 days of the NT diet, my blood pressure has dropped 40 pts. I was getting readings of 200/160, and yesterday I had 123 over 73. Still spikes, but is dropping steadily.

Unbelievable.

I never believed I was a carb person, and have been avoiding them for years, still gaining weight. Steady increase in blood pressure, despite eating healthy, organic foods.

And who would have thought the order in which you eat them matters. I always craved bread and potatoes more than dessert. I'm in heaven finishing a meal with a red potato, or following egg for breakfast with flax wheat toast. And the fog is clearing. Still waiting to see a weight drop, but the blood pressure change is amazing!"

—Mieltje, Deer Park, IL 🙠

Optimal Meal Ideas for Carb Types

Carb types can use these ideal meal suggestions to get started.

- For breakfast, start with a fresh vegetable juice, then have an egg white and vegetable omelet, *or* a cup of freshly cooked oatmeal or other whole grain, topped off with fresh apple slices and cinnamon. As an option, you can add in a raw egg white while the cereal is still hot (the heat from the cereal will be enough to properly cook the egg white).

- Have a Carb Type breakfast shake made by blending 4-6 ounces of reduced-fat milk or plain low-fat yogurt, 1/2 cup to 1 cup of fresh fruit, 1 whole raw egg and 1 teaspoon of unheated, raw honey.

- For lunch, start with another fresh vegetable juice, then have a salad with some low-fat cheese or cottage cheese and/or a dressing made with low-fat plain yogurt as your source of protein (flavor the plain yogurt with fresh chives or fresh dill).

- Another idea for lunch, start with a fresh vegetable juice, followed by a sandwich made with sliced turkey or chicken breast with lettuce, tomato, onion and mustard on slices of whole sprouted-grain or sourdough bread. If desired, have some fresh, organic corn on the cob to finish your meal.

- For dinner, start with fresh vegetable juice, then have another salad with some chicken breast, turkey breast, Cornish hen, light-colored fish or ostrich as your source of protein, or have a serving of Carb Type chicken vegetable soup (recipe below). If desired, finish this meal with a slice of whole sprouted-grain or sourdough bread or a small baked potato with a small amount of olive oil or butter.

Prime Carb Type Juicing Recipes

- **Each serving size of juice should be between 8 and 16 ounces**

- **At least two-thirds of every juice should be made with very-low-carb and/or low-carb vegetables (see the Carb Type food chart for vegetable classification).**

1. Cucumber, tomato & zucchini with some lemon & lime

2. Cucumber, romaine lettuce & zucchini with some lemon & lime

3. Cucumber, romaine lettuce, a whole beet (with the stems & leaves), plus some carrot & apple

4. Cucumber, red & green leaf lettuce, parsley & a kiwi

5. Cucumber, romaine lettuce, parsley & pineapple

6. Cherry tomatoes, bell pepper, parsley & lime

7. Green cabbage, green leaf lettuce, carrot & apple

8. Cucumber, romaine lettuce, carrot & apple

9. Tomato, bell pepper, parsley, kale, carrot & apple

10. Red or green cabbage, broccoli (the stem, not the tops), carrot & apple

11. Romaine lettuce, fennel, carrot, ginger root & fresh mint leaves

12. Tomato, bell pepper, parsley, kale, garlic, ginger root, lemon & lime. (This is the 'protection recipe' and it is especially good for strengthening immune system activity.)

In cold weather feel free to add some fresh ginger root to every juice recipe. Ginger root is well known to be a 'warming' herb.

Carb Type Chicken Vegetable Soup recipe #1
(for lunch and/or dinner)

Ingredients:

- 2 quarts of spring or filtered water
- 4 organic or free-range chicken breasts with the bones & skin
- 3 medium-size organic red or yellow onions, peeled, sliced & diced
- 3 cloves of organic garlic, peeled & diced
- 1 inch of freshly grated organic ginger root
- 6 medium-size organic carrots, sliced & diced (buy the bunch carrots with the green tops, but don't put the green tops in the soup)
- 2 medium-size organic zucchinis, sliced & diced
- 1 medium-size bunch of organic parsley, chopped
- 2 cups of organic tomatoes, sliced & diced

Method:

- Pour the water into a large glass or stainless steel pot. Add the chicken breast, onions, garlic, ginger root, carrots & zucchinis.

- Cover & cook on simmer for 5 to 6 hours. Turn off the heat.

- Now, stir the parsley and tomatoes thoroughly into the soup. Put the cover back on the pot and let the soup sit for 1 hour.

- Remove the chicken breast from the soup, take the skin off the breast and take the chicken meat off the bones. Discard the skin and bones.

- Chop up the chicken meat and add this back to the soup. Stir and then ladle the soup into a bowl and serve moderately hot.

Enjoy this delicious prime Carb Type nourishment!

The Essential NT Guidelines: Mixed Types

If you are a mixed type you have lots of good news. If you are this type you have the broadest selection of food available to you. Your primary concern will be to make sure you appropriately combine your protein and carb food types.

Traditional metabolic typing does not appreciate this and this was one of the largest frustrations we had with it. Mixed types in the old system was simply did not seem to do as well as protein or carb types.

However after a few years of working with the Metabolic Typing we realized this relative lack of response was largely related to improper combination of their protein and carb type foods. Once we incorporated this simple change we noticed the same type of radical improvements for mixed type individuals as protein and carb types.

Mixed types have very broad nutritional needs. They need foods that are right for both Protein Types and Carb Types. They typically gravitate toward eating a large variety of foods, and eating a large variety of foods IS most important for a Mixed Type. Mixed Types can eat high-quality sources of protein and fat together with very-low-carb or low-carb vegetables very freely, but they need to be careful with their intake of high-carb foods.

Mixed Types can identify with many of the characteristics that both Protein Types and Carb Types are familiar with—but Mixed Types do not experience these characteristics as intensely as Protein Types or Carb Types. They feel very good with, and thus gravitate toward, eating meat and vegetable type meals such as a salad with meat or fish, chicken vegetable soup or beef stew.

The classic "balanced" meal that is so commonly advocated for everyone actually works best for Mixed Types.

The table for mixed type foods is not easily displayed in this book format so it is freely available at my web site: You will also find a link on that page that allows you to take the computerized nutritional typing test that can help you identify which nutritional type you are.

Mercola.com/MixedType

Hypothyroid and High Blood Pressure Improves

Lou had a history of high blood pressure and low thyroid function. He developed hypertension about five years ago, and he was shown to have a thyroid problem a year earlier.

He has been on Synthroid since August 2005, which was able to reduce his fatigue and brain fog.

He exercises religiously and has competed in two Iron Man competitions. His initial NT assessment in November 2005 found him to be a Carb Type. For over 10 weeks he faithfully followed the prime Carb Type meal plan and he experienced significant improvement in his energy and stamina.

Additionally, he had no cravings and was able to go four to six hours in between meals before he felt the need to eat again. However, he eventually began to feel a need to increase his intake of raw butter and felt less satisfied with his Carb-Type meals. He tried some raw red meat, which he enjoyed and found to be very satisfying.

Around the same time, he increased the frequency, intensity and duration of his exercise and stopped taking his medication for hypertension, and amazingly his thyroid disease remarkably improved. In February 2006, Lou repeated his NT assessment and in his second report, he was re-assessed as a protein type.

At this point, it was clear that Lou was initially only a functional Carb Type and now he may only be a functional Protein Type. Time will tell, but it is likely that he is a Mixed Type. At this time, Lou continues to feel very good eating an almost all raw food version of the prime Protein Type meal plan. His energy is good and his blood pressure has been in a healthier range. He recently completed a half Iron Man competition and felt very strong doing so.

—*Lou, Santa Barbara, California* ⮞

The Prime Mixed Type Meal Plan Guidelines

Mixed Types should follow these guidelines to achieve optimal health.

1. Make a commitment to choose *all* of your foods from the Mixed Type primary and secondary food charts following these guidelines. Mixed Types should eat foods that are right for both Protein Types and Carb Types at every meal.

2. Give faithful attention to food quality. Eat fresh, organic food as often as possible and consider what you will eat raw and what you will eat cooked. When cooking, never overcook your food. Use low-temperature cooking as often as you can, and, ideally, only eating meats from healthy, humanely raised organic animals.

3. The prime Mixed Type meal plan is based on starting *every meal* with high-quality proteins and fat together with vegetable nutrition selected from the Primary Foods Chart. These foods are printed in green, blue and brown, and they are your most metabolically important foods. Always consume your most metabolically important foods *first at every meal*.

4. From the food choices available on the Mixed Type Primary Foods Chart, create the foundation for each one of your meals with faithful attention to the following Mixed Type food-combining guidelines:

- Proteins printed in green (Protein Type protein) should be eaten with vegetables printed in green, which are Carb Type vegetables.

- Proteins printed in blue (Carb Type protein) should be eaten with vegetables printed in blue (Protein Type vegetables).

- Eating a protein that is printed in green plus a protein that is printed in blue, together with at least one vegetable printed in green and at least one vegetable printed in blue, *and* some additional high-quality fat or oil printed in brown, is the *Mixed Type meal ideal*. This sounds confusing, but trust me, you will get the hang of it quickly—and your body will thank you for the effort.

5. Focus on implementing the Mixed Type meal ideal as often as you can and eat consciously! Pay attention to what you are eating and if you do not already do so, then begin to practice eating slowly and chewing your food thoroughly. As for how much protein, how many vegetables and how much additional fat or oil you should eat–initially, let your appetite be your guide. Listen to your body, trust what it tells you and learn from your experience!

6. When eating breakfast, lunch and dinner, any of the foods on the Secondary Foods Chart may be eaten—but only after you have completely finished your Primary Foods.

7. If you need a snack in between meals, choose your snack from the Primary Foods Chart and/or from the nuts and seeds that are on the Secondary Foods Chart. (This includes nut butters such as almond butter and seed butters such as tahini.) The foods printed in both orange and red on the Secondary Foods Chart, including the sweet fruits, are not appropriate for between-meal snacks.

TAKE CONTROL

Rare Childhood Disease Improves Dramatically

Krista was 4 years old when she visited our clinic and had been diagnosed with Angelman's Syndrome, which is a relatively rare disease. Children with this have a stiff, jerky gait, absent speech, excessive laughter and seizures. Krista also had irregular heartbeats.

It is common for conventional medicine to develop very precise diagnostic criteria for relatively exotic symptom combinations that result from not following natural medical approaches. They have no clue what to attribute the cause to and are equally clueless about solutions.

About the only solace they provide to patients with these conditions is a worthless label.

Krista's Mom, Karen, began feeding her a gluten/casein-free diet and she immediately slept better, her diaper rash cleared up, her cognitive function improved and her staring spells diminished.

However, Krista continued to experience a number of other physical and behavioral symptoms that indicated severe underlying metabolic imbalance. Her NT test showed that she was a Protein Type.

Krista continued to engage in aggressive behavior (kicking, biting, slapping, pulling hair) until it was discovered that she was intolerant to any food that comes from a cow—even raw dairy. Avoiding all cow-derived foods helped to improve Krista's behavior.

Also, Karen has been feeding Krista raw bison, raw salmon and raw eggs, and she reports that overall Krista's progress has been "fabulous." She has seen amazing improvement in Krista's cognitive and learning abilities.

Krista has been talking, which was amazing in light of the fact that doctors had previously told Karen that Krista would never be able to talk. She also has more awareness, seeks to be more involved in activities and has learned to ride a bike. She no longer has constipation and eczema. Additionally, she is no longer intolerant to beef.

This is an absolute amazing testimony to the power of natural foods that are right for a child's Nutritional Type. Application of very simple approaches has resulted in dramatic improvements in a condition that is generally regarded as hopeless in conventional medicine.

—Krista, Mount Pleasant, Michigan ॐ

Optimal Meal Ideas for Mixed Types

Here are some examples of prime meals for Mixed Types.

Breakfast:

If you have a light appetite, have 8 ounces of fresh vegetable juice made with celery and spinach or asparagus, mixed together with 1 raw egg and 1 or 2 tablespoons of raw cream. Or, have some cottage cheese mixed with grated cauliflower or with chopped celery and spinach, mixed together with high-lignan flaxseed oil.

- If you have a stronger appetite for breakfast, have a chicken or turkey salad made with both the white and dark meat, together with a mix of chopped celery, tomato, parsley, scallion and one or two tablespoons of olive oil or raw cream (instead of mayonnaise). Serve this on a bed of romaine lettuce.

- If desired, either of the above breakfasts can be finished with an apple or pear slathered with raw almond butter or simply have some fresh fruit by itself.

Lunch:

- Mix together sliced roast beef and grated raw cheese with chopped bell pepper, mushroom, onion and olive oil.

- Have sliced salmon or salmon tartar with a lettuce salad that includes cherry tomatoes, cucumber and avocado. Drizzle olive oil on top if desired.

- Wrap slices of turkey breast or ham around celery stalks and then dip into raw sour cream or fresh cream. (Mix some fresh herbs, such as chives or dill, into the cream.)

- Have some steak tartar or a rare and juicy burger on a bed of lettuce, tomato and onion (without the bun, of course).

- If desired, any of the above lunches can be finished with a small serving of fresh fruit mixed into a small serving of raw kefir or raw yogurt.

Dinner:

- Start with a small baby, organic spinach salad that includes asparagus tips, sliced mushroom caps, fresh dill, olive oil and the cheese of your choice. Then, choose any one of the following Mixed Type meal ideas for your main course:
   o Have steak tartar or a rare and juicy steak plus an egg, together with chopped bell pepper, mush-rooms, onions and olive oil.

o Have a chicken thigh with some sablefish or tilapia together with steamed broccoli, kale, leek and cauli-flower. Put some raw butter on the vegetables.

- Familiar food combinations such as chicken vegetable soup or turkey vegetable soup (without noodles), beef stew or lamb stew (without carrots and potatoes), and chili (without the beans) are all recommended for Mixed Types not only at dinner, but *for any meal.*

- If desired, finish any of the above dinners with an "after-dinner cocktail" of 6-8 ounces of fresh, organic vegetable juice, or, if you feel a need for some starchy carbohydrates, have a small serving of wild rice eaten with walnuts and high-lignan flaxseed oil or a baked potato with raw butter.

Keeping Track of Your Body's Responses to Your New Meal Plan

When you first start eating right for your Nutritional Type, you'll want to pay careful attention to how your body is responding to the foods you're eating. This will eventually become second-nature to you, but in the beginning we recommend using the tool that we have developed called: "Learning to Listen to Your Body." You can find these tables online at takecontrolofyourhealth.com/listentoyourbody.

This is a systematic and simple way to assess your response to your nutrition plan. Similar to a diary, The "Learning to Listen to your Body" sheets will help you learn from your experience and discover for yourself what is right for you.

And, remember, once you learn the guidelines that are right for you, and experience how your body feels, you'll find that NT is an incredibly healthy way to eat for the rest of your life that, importantly, is not difficult and doesn't require burdensome effort.

Can Your Nutritional Type Change?

Your type can, in fact, change. However, for most people, once your Nutritional Type is correctly identified, it does not change.

As far as your NT changing, this is a matter of the difference between what we refer to as your "genetic type," or the NT that you were born with, and your "functional type"—the NT that you are simply functioning at today.

Occasionally your genetic type can weaken, and as a result you can move into a different NT pattern. This may be caused by:

- Eating the wrong foods for your Nutritional Type

- Stress

- Environmental factors such as seasonal changes

If this occurs after you start balancing your body chemistry, it is possible that you may move back and forth between your genetic and functional types. Until the strength is restored in your body, you may, therefore, move into different Nutritional Types.

However, if your genetic type is the same as your functioning type (and this is the case with most people), then your NT will most likely never change.

Either way, a change in your NT is not something you need to worry about. You simply follow your program and retest occasionally to check on your Nutritional Type and see how you're doing. When you follow your NT, things just work out in a very natural way.

What if I'm a Vegetarian and a Protein Type?

People who follow a vegetarian diet are often concerned about changing their eating habits if they turn out to be Protein Types. Unfortunately, some of the most seriously ill patients I have seen are people who are Protein Types clinging to the belief that they need to be a vegetarian. They are relying on their brain to help them select foods rather than listening to the powerful intuitive clues their body is providing them in essential feedback loops to help them improve their health.

This is because Protein Types need to eat high-purine animal protein in order to be achieve optimal health. The whole point of NT is to identify what foods are right for your specific and unique biochemistry, and that goes far beyond any theory or belief. NT has to do with what is right for your genes, and what is right from a genetic standpoint in terms of the kinds of foods and kinds of nutrients that are right for your metabolism.

While being vegetarian might be a choice that benefits some people, it is a choice that is NOT conducive to health for Protein Types. People in this group tend to suffer terribly by developing numerous health problems and never achieving the level of health they are seeking if they choose to remain on a vegetarian diet.

I'm Having Problems With Digestion . . . What do I Do?

In order to benefit from eating the right foods for your Nutritional Type, you must be able to digest your food properly. Your body, however, may be damaged and not able to produce the hydrochloric acid and enzymes necessary to properly digest your food.

If you are eating the foods that are right for your Nutritional Type, yet are having digestive problems such as:

- Belching or burping
- Food seeming like it's sitting like a rock in your stomach and just not moving through
- Your digestion seems unusually slow
- You have heartburn or intestinal gas
- Any other signs of indigestion

. . . Remember to **eat consciously!** Pay attention to what you are eating and if you do not already do so, begin to practice eating slowly and chewing your food thoroughly.

It is also important to eat your food under calm conditions. You shouldn't be watching upsetting news on TV, having an argument with someone, or worrying about a problem that you're dealing with while you eat. This is because stressful situations such as these will shut off the digestive process and make it much more difficult for you to digest your food.

You may also benefit from taking some hydrochloric acid and/or enzyme supplements with your meals to help your digestive process. Taking a daily probiotic is also recommended. When taking supplements, you should seek an experienced natural medical clinician to guide you through the process.

Why Taking Supplements Can be Dangerous if you Don't Know Your NT

I'm very much opposed to the indiscriminate use of supplements, as they can cause far more harm than good. Foods can be wonderful for you if they are right for your Nutritional Type, but the challenging point for many to accept is that even locally biodynamically grown organic vegetables can be bad for you if they're wrong for your Nutritional Type. And when you apply that notion to a disease process, such as heart disease or high cholesterol, if you eat the wrong foods for your Nutritional Type you may increase your heart disease or bad cholesterol, even if those foods don't contain cholesterol.

Foods are good or bad for you, depending upon what's right for your Nutritional Type, and the identical scenario is also true for supplements. Vitamins and minerals have specific effects on your metabolism, so to simply start taking supplements because you read about them in an article or you hear friends say that it was good for them, is actually an unwise and potentially unhealthy thing to do. We do not recommend doing that.

Taking an individual nutrient or multivitamin that is wrong for your NT can cause or worsen an imbalance in your biochemistry.

When Will I Experience the Benefits of Nutritional Typing?

Most people will start to notice benefits of eating the right foods for their NT within the first few weeks. However, it is important to appreciate that you will continue to realize your full health potential over time.

If you are suffering from a degenerative process, you should give yourself a few years of really being faithful to the program. At the end of that time, when you look back you'll be amazed at the changes that have taken place in your body, just by eating the right foods—and stopping the wrong ones—for your Nutritional Type.

Nutritional Typing Success Stories

Those who use Nutritional Typing are often amazed at the profound benefits they experience. Here we've compiled just a small sampling of tremendous improvements that people have experienced from NT.

How Do I Find Out My Nutritional Type?

All of our patients at the Optimal Wellness Center (my health clinic just outside of Chicago) were required to take the computerized Metabolic Typing analysis as part of their evaluation in our clinic. The cost for that analysis, with a one-hour follow-up consultation with a therapist, was $180 (this was typically reimbursed by third-party insurance companies).

However, the high price of the analysis has prevented many people from taking this valuable test, which we believe should be available to everyone. A portion of that fee went to pay for the actual computerized test that was developed by Bill Wolcott.

To provide a less-expensive alternative, we've developed a simpler, much more affordable test to nutritionally type you and an online evaluation and support forum, which is moderated by one of the nutritionists that works in our clinic.

So we now can finally offer the test to our online subscribers All you need to do is go to:

Mercola.com/NT

The test also includes participation for one month in our online forum so you can access the thousands of questions that people have already written and also have a full month of free one on one coaching with our Nutritional Typing coaches.

We are extremely excited to be able to offer the NT program, as those who apply its principles experience phenomenal health benefits. Give it a try for yourself, and experience for the first time what truly optimal health really feels like.

Grains and Sugars—
The Villans In The Obesity Epidemic

**Ninety percent of the money that Americans spend
on food is for processed food!**

This is the crux of our diabetes and obesity epidemic. People are simply exchanging convenience and taste for health.

It might change in the future, but for the time being and likely in the lifetime of everyone reading this, you have a genetic requirement to consume whole, unprocessed foods. This means someone needs to spend time in the kitchen to produce healthy food, as it is unavailable at nearly all commercial restaurants.

> Your ancestors consumed nothing but whole foods found in nature, and this is what your body is designed to eat.

Large scale processing of food is only about 100 years old, but this processing is one of the primary reasons that we have an epidemic of chronic diseases.

Diabetes Or Pre-Diabetes Now Affects *One In Three* Americans

One in three! If this doesn't qualify as an epidemic, I surely don't know what does. Just let this statistic hit home and reflect on it for a short while. One out of every three people you know has this problem. This is mind-boggling. Diabetes can cause early death, blindness, kidney failure, heart attacks, very painful nerve damage, and is the most common reason people have their legs amputated.

But this epidemic could be virtually eliminated overnight. Avoiding processed foods and exercising are two of the primary ways by which diabetes can be prevented and, in many cases, reversed. But another important technique is to limit grains until your insulin balance comes under control again.

TAKE CONTROL

Cut His Blood Sugar Readings in Half

"At the time I started reading your articles, my blood sugar reading was between 220 and 300. I cut out the grains, dairy products, and the high carbohydrate suppliers like rice, pasta and potatoes. I started using the advice from your website and in less than a week my blood sugar dropped to 150 and is continuing to fall."

—*Graham Kemshell, London, United Kingdom* ❧

His Cholesterol Dropped 80 Points

I found out about Dr. Mercola's Take Control of Your Health program through my family doctor, who told me that he personally follows Dr. Mercola's dietary guidelines and recommended it for my husband and me. My husband lost 25 lbs in 4 months, and his cholesterol went down 80 points!

—*Lynette White, Ahwahnee, California* ❧

The Solution to Controlling Your Weight Is Simple

The diabetic epidemic is clearly a major problem, because it has such devastating consequences. But it is no mystery that we also have an obesity epidemic in the United States. Not only do one in three people have diabetes or pre-diabetes, but in addition, **one in three are obese**—not simply overweight, but obese.

Another one in three Americans are overweight, for a total of two out of three Americans all told who are above a healthy weight. Fortunately, the steps that would eliminate diabetes also serve to normalize weight. Most people believe that the solution is simply to limit your calories and increase your exercise, but this approach is too simplistic and does not actually work for most people.

Exercise is another critical element of the weight-control equation, but not because it burns the extra calories you are consuming. Exercise does help you increase your metabolic rate to burn more calories, but it also helps to normalize the hormones insulin and leptin, both of which have a huge effect on weight control.

As discussed in Chapter Two on Nutritional Typing, it is *not the total calories* you eat, but the ratio of proteins, fats and carbs you were genetically designed to eat that is the key factor. And for many, especially those who thrive on a high-protein diet, reducing your intake of grains is essential.

Not All Carbs Are Created Equal

Avoiding grains and sugars has been popularized by Dr. Atkin's low-carbohydrate diet. Although low-carb dieting is frequently effective for weight loss, especially for protein types, the low-carb diet is still a one-size-fits-all approach that misses the fact that every individual has varying needs for the optimal amount and type of carbohydrates, proteins and fats in their diet all depending on their nutritional type.

There are different types of carbohydrates, and the ones that should compose the majority of your carbohydrate intake are found mostly in high-fiber vegetables that grow above the ground. Your body prefers these complex carbohydrates, because they slow the release of simple carbohydrates, like glucose, and do not cause a significant increase in your insulin levels. Insulin is the fat-building hormone in the body; therefore, increases in insulin cause weight gain.

On the other hand, there are potentially "troublesome" carbohydrates that you need to reduce or eliminate from your diet, and they are found in grains, sugars, and sugary foods, as well as starchy vegetables like potatoes, corn (actually a grain), carrots and beets. These carbohydrates will increase your insulin levels and tend to promote weight gain and illness.

You Are What THEY Ate

For hundreds of generations, your ancestors existed primarily on a diet of wild animals and vegetation. It was only with the advent of agriculture a mere 6,000 years ago—an extraordinarily small period in time—that humans began eating large amounts of sugar and starch in the form of grains and potatoes in their diets. Indeed, **your genetic code was set before the advent of agriculture**; so, in biological terms, our bodies are still those of hunter-gatherers.

While the shift to agriculture produced other indisputable gains for man, societies which transitioned from a primarily meat/vegetation diet to one high in grains consistently show a reduced lifespan and stature, increases in infant mortality and infectious disease, and higher nutritional deficiencies. This is because consuming sugar also impairs your white blood cells' function and thereby decreases your body's immune system, making you more vulnerable to disease. Keep in mind that these ancient societies used entirely unrefined and organic grains. Today over 95% of grains consumed in the United States are highly processed, making the negative consequences of grains even worse.

The physiology of contemporary humans has not changed much from your distant ancestors, and your body has never adapted to the excessive amount of carbohydrates from grains and sweets in the present-day diet. In fact, we live in a nation whose diet is still largely based on the seriously conflicted and misguided USDA Food Pyramid, which recommends an unhealthy 6–11 servings of breads, cereals, rice, and pasta per day. This surplus of insulin-spiking carbohydrates is one of the primary reasons for the obesity epidemic and the scourge of related chronic diseases like diabetes, heart disease, cancer, and Alzheimer's.

It is important to understand that it is primarily your body's response to the overindulgence of grain and sugars, not your intake of fat, which makes you fat. Your body has a limited capacity to *store* carbohydrates, but it can easily *convert* those excess carbohydrates, via insulin, into body fat, which means the more carbohydrates you eat, the more body fat you'll have. When a government agency recommends the consumption of 6–11 servings of grains per day, plus four servings of fruit, which is also high in simple sugars, it becomes quite obvious what the inevitable and observed consequences will be—a nation of overweight people.

The fact is that any meal or snack high in carbohydrates from grains or sweets generates a rapid rise in blood glucose. To adjust for this rise, your pancreas secretes the hormone insulin into your bloodstream, which lowers your blood sugar. Insulin is essentially a storage hormone, developed over thousands of years to help you store the excess calories from carbohydrates in the form of fat in case of famine.

Throughout most of human history, and certainly in many areas of the world today, there were frequent periods of mass starvation caused by droughts and other natural disasters that depleted the availability of vegetation, containing the complex carbohydrates that are the carbs you should eat, and therefore the game animals that relied on this vegetation. Adaptation gradually developed defenses against this starvation so your body could convert any excess carbohydrates to fat so fat stores could be used for energy over time. You are, in other words, walking around in a body well designed to pull you through potential starvation. The problem is, you live in a time and a place with the extreme opposite situation—we don't experience times of famine; instead we have an overabundance of grains, starches, and sweets, and food companies are marketing them endlessly to us.

To make matters even worse, high insulin levels also lower two other important hormones—glucagon and growth hormone—that are responsible for *burning* fat and sugar and promoting muscle development. In other words, insulin produced from consuming excess carbohydrates found in grains and sugars promotes fat, and then wards off your body's ability to lose that fat and build muscle!

Additionally, another action of insulin is that it *causes* you to be hungry, and it's usually a craving for sweets. As your blood sugar increases following a carbohydrate meal, your pancreas secretes insulin to lower your blood sugar. This lowered blood sugar results in hunger, frequently less than a couple of hours after the meal with the excessive carbs. If ignored long enough, this hunger may cause you to feel ravenous and ready to "crash" as a result of hypoglycemia or low blood sugar. In order to raise your blood sugars, your body will naturally crave high sugar foods like sweets or grains, which lead to a vicious roller coaster ride of high and low blood sugars. The roller coaster may cause you to become a sugar and grain addict, and this causes you to become increasingly fatter, fatigued, depressed, and sick.

TAKE CONTROL

Arthritis Gone and Mentally Sharper, Too!

"I am 54 years old. About twenty years ago, I developed pain in my knees. The pain eventually spread to my back, neck and hands. It was chronic. Doctors told me it was due to age and wear and tear. They concluded there was nothing I could do about it except to take pills and eventually get surgery. Since I am not overweight, no one, not even I, suspected that my diet which consisted heavily of breads, cereals, cakes and sweets had anything to do with my condition.

About a year ago, I received Dr. Mercola's newsletter and read how grains can have a negative impact on one's health. I decided to gradually start removing grain-based foods from my diet. It was also hard, because I was especially addicted to the breads and cakes. After a short time, I noticed a diminishing of the pain in my knees.

Encouraged by my improvement, I decided to attack the condition head-on and ordered Dr. Mercola's Take Control of Your Health program. I quickly found how to eat right and exercise right. In the months that I have been following Dr. Mercola's program, I have become noticeably leaner (according to co-workers) and my aches and pains have all but disappeared. One improvement that I did not expect is that I am in a constant state of mental sharpness. I am more alert, never sluggish, and my attention span has greatly improved. And I'm just getting started!"

—*Dominick Crupi, Glendale, NY* ❧

Now back to the good news. You have this book, and it provides you with a practical solution. By eating according to your unique and specific nutritional type (discussed in Chapter Two), you'll find the craving for these unhealthy but tempting foods disappears relatively quickly.

Who Needs to Limit or Eliminate Grains Temporarily?

Those with celiac disease and gluten sensitivities have an obvious additional need to avoid grains, particularly gluten which is found in wheat, spelt, rye, barley, and oats. For those with diabetes and other signs of elevated insulin, such as obesity, high blood pressure or high cholesterol, it is crucial to eliminate grains and sugars. But even people who do not show these obvious signs may need to reduce their grain intake. So, who else should?

Understanding the answer to this question is a central component of successfully applying the Take Control of Your Health program. Fortunately, there is a very precise way to answer this question, and it involves a simple biochemical measurement.

One of the central precepts of Take Control of Your Health is to understand that your body has enormous wisdom and will guide you to the proper healing path if you are sensitive to its signals and integrate its feedback loop into your life. It will be vital for you to learn to pay attention to this feedback in terms of the symptoms you have, physical signs and laboratory testing if you are to achieve optimal health.

Because of the epidemic of abnormal insulin levels in the United States, one of lab tests that we have all our patients do is a fasting blood test for insulin which you can get at your physician's office. The following table shows the insulin levels and how to interpret them. The only requirement for this test is that you are fasting when the blood sample is drawn. That means nothing to eat or drink except water for 8 hours, or ideally 12 hours, before the test.

Insulin Level mcU/mL	
0-3	Excellent and good glycemic control
3-5	Very good control, but room for improvement
5-10	Impaired—heading for serious problems
>10	Out of control—in serious need of change

So, if your insulin level is above 5, the odds are highly likely that your health would improve by vastly reducing grains—and yes, that means even whole, unprocessed grains.

Corn Is NOT A Vegetable

Most people can easily name the common grains such as rice, wheat, oats, barley, and rye, but forget that corn also belongs in that category, as they perceive corn to be a vegetable.

Corn is a grain. It has all the negative health impacts of a grain. Its processing into high fructose corn syrup is responsible for much of our obesity epidemic. High-fructose corn syrup, primarily in sodas, is now the number one source of calories for Americans. The average American drinks an estimated 56 gallons of soda each year. **That's an average of 600 cans of soda per person, per year.**

According to recent research, the demise of certain Native American tribes in earlier centuries can be mainly attributed to corn. With the arrival of the Spanish, their eating patterns shifted away from the primarily meat and vegetation diet of a hunter-gatherer society to a homogenous diet based almost entirely on corn. The research shows that the bones of the Native Americans during and after this transition show much higher evidence of anemia, dental cavities, osteoarthritis, infections and other health issues than those who lived prior to this transition.

Corn is relatively high in sugar, which is one of the main reasons it's America's number one crop, consuming over 80 million acres of

U.S. land and sneaking its way into an endless array of food (and other) products.

It is also important to understand that corn is second only to soybeans as the most genetically modified (GMO) crop in the United States GMOs, which were first introduced in 1995, are a potential disaster waiting to happen, as no studies have been done with humans to show what happens when genetically modified foods are consumed.

Sugar, The Challenge to Taking Control of Your Health

Most people are addicted to sugar. Along with grain addiction, the over-consumption of added sugars—such as high-fructose corn syrup, fructose, glucose, dextrose, or sucrose (table sugar)—is one of the major health problems facing our nation today.

For just a *partial* idea of the ill health effects of excess sugar consumption, consider that sugar has been cited as a contributing factor to:

—Overweight and obesity

—Immune system suppression, inviting infection and disease

—Premature aging

—Cancer of the breast, ovaries, prostate, and rectum

—Decreased absorption of calcium and magnesium

—Diabetes

—Fatigue

—Decreased energy and reduced ability to build muscle

—Heart disease

—Crohn's disease and ulcerative colitis

—Osteoporosis

—Yeast infections

—Depression

—Dental decay and gum disease

Sugars are simple carbohydrates processed by your body in the same manner as grains. That is, any excess sugars in your body are converted by insulin and subsequently into fat—and just like grains, Americans are consuming an enormous quantity of sugar. In the past two decades in the United States, sugar consumption has increased by over 30%. In fact, the average per-person sugar intake is now 175 pounds per year! That's 300,000 calories per year, or 800 calories per day, from sugar!

This is asking for serious health trouble even by the ill-advised USDA standards, which states that the average American can eat up to 10 teaspoons of added sugars per day as a part of their 2,000 daily calories. Unfortunately, the average American is consuming well over 3,000 calories per day, including over 20 teaspoons of added sugars.

The most common form of sugar intake is soda. Therefore, eliminating soda is one of the most important steps you can take to improve your physical health. If you are unable to achieve this by yourself, I would strongly encourage you to go to my website and type in "Turbo Tapping" in the search box; you will find an article that gives you a simple energy psychology technique that is highly effective at stopping this devastating addiction.

TAKE CONTROL

She Had No Idea How Addicted to Sugar Her Family Was . . .

"I work for a chiropractor and he taught me a lot about health and wellness. I heard him, but for some reason it didn't truly sink in until I heard Dr. Mercola speak at a seminar in Chicago.

I realized how my eating habits were killing me—and worse yet—killing my children. I purchased Dr. Mercola's Take Control of Your Health Program. By the time I got home, I knew my nutritional type and was ready to clean out the cupboards and start on the road to recovery.

My husband and children thought I had gone crazy! I had no idea how addicted to sugar my family was! Now, my children are never sick and they are going to grow up with healthy eating habits. I was so proud—and a little shocked—when my 5 year old daughter turned down a sucker when one was offered to her by a teller at a bank. My children seem to have more energy than other kids when playing sports.

We are far from perfect, but we have come a long way and are learning and doing better each day. It's never too late to change for the better. I am a faithful reader of Dr. Mercola's newsletter. I often forward articles to friends and family who need advice about health and print out articles to leave in the reception area at my chiropractic office. I am very grateful to Dr. Mercola for sharing his knowledge."

—*Rachel Smith, New Castle, IN* ❧

In addition to soda, there are high-sugar culprits disguised as "healthy" by food marketers like: "fruit drinks," "fruit beverages," and "fruit punch," such as Snapple, which contain anywhere from 1% to 40% of fruit juice, but all of which contain loads of sugar, usually high-fructose corn syrup.

> **For many people, sugar is an authentic addiction similar to cigarette dependency,** but it affects your health even more severely. Although some would disagree with my position, because they fail to appreciate the enormous influence insulin levels have on virtually every chronic disease, including cancer. The solution is not to keep hunting for ways to "safely" maintain the addiction, such as with artificial sweeteners. The solution is to overcome the addiction.

Even the sugars in 100% real fruit juice can quickly add up: real fruit juice, whether store-bought or freshly squeezed, has about eight full teaspoons of sugar per eight-ounce glass. This sugar is typically a fruit sugar called fructose, which is every bit as dangerous as the regular table sugar sucrose, since it also causes a major increase in insulin levels.

This doesn't mean that you should avoid fruit, just fruit juice. When the fruit is intact and whole, its fiber will moderate the release of fructose and secondarily insulin into your bloodstream. However, if you are overweight, have high blood pressure or have high blood sugar levels, you would be wise to avoid most fruits and just stick with vegetable carbohydrates until you have these problems under control. This is especially true if you are a Protein Nutritional Type. Carbohydrate types are generally better designed to handle the carbohydrates in fruits, especially citrus fruits.

Fortunately, you'll find that by adopting the nutrition principles discussed in the book, and utilizing the tools to overcome emotional barriers, you won't have to "fight" the craving, because it will naturally disappear and you'll be on the fast track to optimal health.

The Fats You Should Eat and The Fats You Should Avoid

Do you know the truth about dietary fat?

True or False:

1. Low-fat diets help you lose weight because eating fat causes weight gain.

2. High-fat, saturated fat, and high-cholesterol foods increase blood cholesterol.

3. High cholesterol levels (180 and above) increase risk of heart disease.

4. Substituting butter and lard with polyunsaturated oils, e.g. vegetable oils, will decrease your risk for heart disease.

Our society teaches that all of these statements are true. But you have to understand that the nutrition information that we are given by the media, our physicians, health organizations, the education system, and diet books is mostly wrong! The reason it is wrong is because it is based on what the food manufacturers want you to believe so they can sell their products. Unfortunately, the replacement of natural fat with artificially processed fats in our food supply has had a devastating effect on our health.

Now let's see how you did on the quiz:

(The quiz answers came from the outstanding book *Eat Fat Lose Fat* by Dr. Mary Enig and Sally Fallon.)

1. Low-fat diets help you lose weight because eating fat causes weight gain.

> **FALSE.** People do lose weight on low-fat diets, primarily because they are taking in fewer calories.

It is a myth that when you eat fat, it immediately adds to your fat stores. Actually, when you eat fat, it is used in the numerous vital functions in your body, including hormone synthesis and cell membrane composition. Eating fat doesn't make you fat.

On the other hand, the only function that carbohydrates have in your body is for energy (which you can also get from protein and fat). Any excess carbohydrates that your body does not need for immediate use, are stored as fat. Therefore, if you want to lose weight, you'll want to focus on cutting down on your carbohydrates.

In actuality, eating fat helps you lose weight, especially if you are a protein type, because fat leads to a feeling of satiety (fullness) much more than carbohydrates and protein. On the other hand, you can be pretty hungry on a low-fat diet, especially if you are a protein type. This can then lead to a larger intake of carbohydrates and then weight gain. Weight Watchers, Jenny Craig, and LA Weight Loss are all based on eating a low-fat diet, so it is not surprising that their long-term success rates are poor.

2. High-fat and high-cholesterol foods increase blood cholesterol.

> **FALSE**. The best scientific studies have found no direct connection whatsoever between high cholesterol foods and high cholesterol levels. However, there is research to show that excess carbohydrates and genetic factors can cause high blood cholesterol.

3. High cholesterol levels (180 and above) increase risk of heart disease.

> **FALSE.** The best studies that have been done in this area have proven this statement to be false.

The Framingham Study examined 500 people over 30 years and found very little difference between the cholesterol levels of those who had heart attacks and those who did not. They did, however, find that people whose cholesterol decreased over the 30 years had a higher risk of death than those whose cholesterol had increased.

The International Athersclerosis Project was published is 1968 in the journal Laboratory Investigations. Researchers performed autopsies on 22,000 corpses from around the world and found about the same amount of fatty plaques in the arteries of vegetarians as they did in the heavy meat eaters. There was also no correlation between cholesterol levels and the amount of artery blockage.

Many studies show that women with high cholesterol levels live longer, and that women with very low cholesterol levels had a death rate over five times higher than women with normal or elevated levels.

4. Consumption of polyunsaturated oils (e.g. vegetable oils) will decrease your risk for heart disease.

> **FALSE.** At least as commonly perceived in the public. The statement is technically true if you restrict the oils to omega-3 fats, but the typical polyunsaturated fat statement widely promoted in the media was not referencing omega-3 fats, but rather omega-6 vegetable fats. Vegetable oil manufacturers such as Wesson Oil and Mazola advertised that their oils were healthier for your heart, this has not proven true. What has proven to be true is that a preponderance of omega-6 polyunsaturated oils can actually increase your risk of cancer. See the Omega-6 Fats section below for further information.

The Weight Gain Myth

The belief that eating fat makes you fat is one of the most prevalent myths today, right up there with Santa Claus and the Easter Bunny. If eating fat makes you fat, why did the incidence of obesity dramatically increase during the low-fat craze in the early 1980's?

During the low-fat craze, people were told that they could eat anything as long as it was low-fat. Supermarket shelves burgeoned with low-fat cookies, crackers, bread, frozen entrees, snacks, potato chips, frozen yogurt, etc., and the public filled up on these items because they could eat the high carb foods they loved without the guilt. The USDA's food pyramid base expanded widely just as people's waistlines grew. Eleven servings of grains, cereals, and breads per day was the absurd recommendation that was the impetus for enormous weight gain in America and worldwide. The National Institute of Health spent several hundred million dollars trying to show a correlation between eating fat and getting heart disease. Five major studies were conducted and none of them showed such a link.[1]

Dr. Walter Willett, of the Harvard School of Public Health, Department of Nutrition collected data regarding 300,000 individuals and their eating patterns. He found that the low-fat diet is clearly unhealthy and has contributed to the obesity epidemic.

Why High Quality Fat Is Your Friend

As you will learn in Chapter Two on Nutritional Typing, our individual needs for dietary fat vary widely. Some people may need up to 400% more fat than others. However, we all need some amount of fat. Dietary fat accomplishes many necessary functions, including the following:

- **Slow stomach emptying:** The more fat in the food you eat, the longer it takes to digest, and the longer you will feel full. You can go longer between meals, and you don't need to eat as much when you have fat in your meal.

- **Stick-to-your-ribs food:** Fat content makes food much better tasting and satisfying. Because fatty food stays in your stomach longer than other types of food, there is enough time for a signal to get to your brain, announcing that you are full.

- **Dietary fats are necessary to absorb fat soluble vitamins:** Some vitamins can only be absorbed with enough dietary fat. The fat in your food stimulates your gallbladder to release bile, which in turn breaks down the fat in food as well as the fat-soluble vitamins. These vitamins, including Vitamins D, A, K, and E, require dietary fat to help absorption. It has been found that Vitamin D is your best protection against cancer.[2] Vitamin A provides a powerful boost for the immune system during infections. Vitamin K is essential to regulate the clotting of your blood, and Vitamin E is a great antioxidant for protecting the heart, blood vessels, and other organs. These are only a few of the valuable functions of these vitamins.

- **Fats fuel your energy:** Fats are the longest-lasting source of energy, both for present needs and in storage for future energy needs. In times of fasting or famine, those who have the most fat have the highest likelihood of survival.

- **Dietary fat provides the building blocks for many of your hormones:** Without dietary fat, you could not even make enough hormones to carry out many of your basic bodily functions. Eating fat is necessary for the production of cortisol, testosterone, estrogen, and progesterone, among other hormones.

- **Your cells require dietary fats to optimally function.** Your cells keep you alive because they are able to exchange and transmit biochemical signals. They can do this because of a complicated but efficient envelope around each cell called the phospholipid bilayer, which is mostly made up of fat.

TAKE CONTROL

Increased Her Good Fats to Drop that 15 Pounds

I can't tell you how much I appreciate the life-changing information I have received from the Take Control of Your Health Program. I am currently 58 years old and most of my life, I have battled with that extra 15 pounds or so. Every time I went on a diet, I would reduce the amount of fat intake, feel hungry all of the time and think about food constantly. Once the diet was over, I would start gaining back the weight within a relatively short period of time.

The information I learned from Dr. Mercola's website and the book/program showed me a better way to eat based on my body type. I increased my good fats, increased my intake of healthy protein, eliminated grains and now have eliminated that extra 15 pounds.

The beauty of this is that I feel satisfied and no longer continuously think about food! My weight has stayed off for over a year and I know inside that with this program I no longer have to think of maintaining my ideal weight as a continuing STRUGGLE!! Thank you for changing my life!

—*Gratefully, Kristine Nelson, Roseville, MN* ࿓

Body Fat Is Also Important

- **Fats as necessary padding:** Don't think of fat padding as dead weight. If it weren't for fat padding your organs, they would be much more vulnerable to every little bump from outside your body. Fat cushions and holds your organs in place, keeping them from sagging. Some organs are especially fat-dependent because of the delicate structures that they house. Your brain, for example, is 60% fat.

- **Fat as insulation:** It is hard to maintain a body temperature of 98.6°F when the winter winds blow. Fat insulates you and helps you tolerate the cold and maintain your body temperature so that your enzymes (which are picky about temperature) can work properly.

Dangerous Half-Truths

This does not, however, mean that all fats are good; in fact, some forms of fat are very dangerous. But there is a great deal of confusion and misinformation being spread about the subject, often by sources that seem authoritative. Besides grains and sugars, there is no category of food that the public has received more dangerous half-truths about than edible oils.

To understand just how dangerous this misinformation is, you need to know that **before the 1920s heart attacks did not exist;** but by 1950, heart disease was the cause of 30 percent of all deaths in the U.S. What happened?

Prior to 1910, Americans ate traditional natural foods such as meat, eggs, butter, and cheese. But in 1910, hydrogenated vegetable oils, such as Crisco and margarine, were introduced into the U.S. These were designed to replace lard. Hydrogenation is a process by which the liquid oil is heated at very high temperatures to make it solid, which makes it more stable. The problem with hydrogenating oils is that the process turns the fat into trans fat. The word "trans" refers to the artificial chemical configuration of the fat after it is hydrogenated.

Trans fats are linked to heart disease and cancer, because your body does not know how to process these artificial chemicals. Also, because trans fats lower your levels of "good" cholesterol, they indirectly lead to high "bad" cholesterol levels. Unfortunately,

> " . . . before the 1920's, heart attacks did not exist."

trans fats are now found in most packaged processed foods, such as baked goods, cereals, cookies, crackers, soup mixes, frozen foods, and fried foods like French fries, tortilla chips, and doughnuts. If you want to stay healthy, there's no question you need to avoid trans fats such as margarine, vegetable shortening and products which contain the words "hydrogenated" or "partially hydrogenated."

Over the years, the intake of eggs, lard, and butter sharply decreased while the use of cheap margarine and vegetable oils quadrupled. After World War II (1945), manufacturers began substituting coconut oil and animal fats with hydrogenated oils for a longer shelf life. Some researchers, such as Ancel Keys, tried to warn the public that hydrogenated fats were causing heart disease, but the hydrogenated oil manufacturers launched a public relations campaign that identified saturated fats as the culprit instead.

In the early 1950s, based only on very partial and inconclusive research, several government and other influential health organizations proposed that the conventional diet that included saturated fats from products like butter, meat, and coconut oil was dangerous to the heart. Even at that time, though, many studies contradicted this assumption, and other nations whose diets had a saturated fat intake higher than Americans were not experiencing near the same rate of heart disease—but this information was largely ignored. The food manufacturers of margarine and corn, safflower, sunflower, and other monounsaturated oils took advantage of the misperception, equating saturated fat with pure evil while promoting their products as essential health foods. Wesson, for instance, promoted its cooking oil as good "for your heart's sake."

The general public embraced unsaturated and hydrogenated fats while shunning saturated fats. By the 1970s, this idea (sometimes called "the lipid hypothesis") had become the prevailing explanation for the epidemic of heart disease, despite the fact that there was no evidence to support it.

What's Good About Saturated Fats?

Saturated fats got scapegoated for problems that had nothing to do with fats, simply because they are not as convenient to market, store, and distribute as trans fats.

Saturated fats are highly stable, because all the carbon links are filled or saturated with hydrogen atoms. This keeps saturated fats from going rancid or switching to the trans fat configuration, even under high heat. For this reason, coconut oil is an excellent oil in which to cook your food. Even at high heat it stays stable.

Saturated fats do not increase risk for heart disease. Consider the Masai people of Tanzania. On their diet of meat and milk only (because they consider plants to be poor quality food, fit only for animals), they have the cleanest arteries in the world. They also have low blood cholesterol.[3]

Interestingly, the Masai individuals who migrate to Nairobi and adopt a modern diet of processed carbs and trans fat begin to have some of the atherosclerotic changes that the rest of the world struggles with.

How Trans Fatty Acids Damage Your Heart

Trans fats can plug up your artery walls by stimulating plaque formation. This has become such a serious problem that an estimated 30,000 to 100,000 people in the United States die every year from premature coronary disease due to trans fatty acids.[4]

As was mentioned above, trans fatty acids also raise your "bad" cholesterol (LDL) and lower your "good" cholesterol (HDL). In fact, trans fatty acids are the worst of all foods for unbalancing your cholesterol—raising the bad and lowering the good.[5] These numbers are reversed when trans fatty acids are removed from the diet.[6]

One of the primary reasons for the deadly effects of trans fatty acids is their ability to dramatically increase inflammation and insulin resistance, so much so that it can lead to a pre-diabetic condition called metabolic syndrome.[7] Furthermore, trans fat also alters membrane structure on your cells, which can seriously impair cellular signaling and lead to a host of potentially serious metabolic anomalies. As a result, enzymes do not get activated as they need to and can stop functioning correctly.

Trans Fats and Diabetes

Trans fatty acids make your body less sensitive to insulin, especially if you already have an insulin resistance problem or are diabetic.[8] Eating these artificial molecules on top of refined carbohydrates is asking for trouble and is likely the reason so many people are now either diabetic or pre-diabetic. If a sugar diet is a slow train to diabetes, then a sugar plus trans fats diet puts you on an express train toward diabetes.

Trans Fats And Autoimmune Disease

As previously mentioned, trans fats increase inflammation in your body. In addition to heart disease, this can also lead to auto-immune disease in which your body starts self-destructing.[9]

For example, asthma is a respiratory disease where the primary problem is over-reactive airways. When dust or other allergens hit the airways, asthmatics suddenly feel as if they are being choked and can hardly breathe. Asthma can be life-threatening. It was found that when an expectant mother ate fish during pregnancy, her kids had less of a risk of asthma. This was probably due to the anti-inflammatory fats in the fish. On the other hand, when pregnant women ate more fish sticks, which contain trans fatty acids, their kids had higher rates of asthma. Even though the fish provided some protective effect against asthma, that was more than outweighed by the damaging effects of the trans fatty acids.[10]

Trans Fatty Acids Can Cause Alzheimer's

It was found over a three-year study that Alzheimer's Disease struck more people who had high trans fatty acid intakes than others, in fact 2.4 times as many people.[11] The same researchers found a protective effect of fish against Alzheimer's.

Trans Fatty Acids And Cancer

In one study it was found that those who ate higher amounts of trans fats showed more evidence of oxidative stress and free radicals in their urine.[12] These in turn increase the risk for cancer, especially when unopposed by antioxidant foods.

Omega-6 Fats

Coinciding with the rise of trans fats in the American diet was a vast increase in the consumption of omega-6 fats, as cheap vegetable oils became pervasive. The typical American consumes far too many omega-6 fats in their diet while consuming very low levels of omega-3.

The primary sources of omega-6 are corn, soy, canola, safflower, and sunflower oil; these oils are overabundant in the typical diet, which explains our excess omega-6 levels. Omega-3, meanwhile, is typically found in flaxseed oil, walnut oil, and fish.

The ideal ratio of omega-6 to omega-3 fats is 1:1. Today, though, our ratio of omega-6 to omega-3 averages from 20:1 to 50:1! That spells serious danger for you. This out-of-balance ratio is one of the most serious health issues plaguing contemporary society; excess omega-6 fats can lead to heart disease, cancer, depression, Alzheimer's disease, rheumatoid arthritis, diabetes, ulcerative colitis, Raynaud's disease, and a host of other illnesses.

Due to the overconsumption of omega-6 oils, I encourage you to limit your intake of these oils—such as vegetable oils including corn, safflower, sunflower, canola, sesame, and soybean oil. You most certainly want to avoid cooking with these oils, because trans fats are formed when vegetable oils are heated to high temperatures during regular cooking. In addition to the trans fat and omega-6 issues, these vegetable oils may suppress your immune system; in fact, vegetable oils are emulsified with water and injected in patients who have had organ transplants specifically to suppress their immune system.[13] They can also cause oxidative damage and interfere with normal thyroid function.[14]

Olive Oil

Instead, the two best vegetable oils are coconut oil and extra-virgin olive oil. Olive oil is a monounsaturated fat and is beneficial because it contains vitamins E and A, chlorophyll, magnesium, squalene, and a host of other cardio-protective nutrients. Olive oil possesses these health benefits because it is unrefined and unheated, unlike other oils.

Olive oil has also been shown to reduce the risk of some cancers and rheumatoid arthritis. Additionally, olive oil is an omega-9 fatty acid, and therefore it does not overload the body with omega-6 fats. However, a drawback to olive oil is that it is more susceptible to oxidative damage than coconut oil when cooked since it is a monounsaturated fat. The best bet with olive oil is to use it on salads, and use coconut oil for your cooking.

Coconut Oil

Coconut oil is a saturated fat that is, I believe, the best oil for cooking due to its better stability at high temperatures. Coconut oil can also help you prevent and fight many diseases and illnesses.[15] And, despite being a saturated fat, it can actually contribute to weight loss.[16]

Coconut oil is particularly recommended for those with diabetes. It helps regulate your blood sugar, thus decreasing the risk of diabetes, or if you have diabetes, lessening the effects of the disease.[17] It also helps raise your metabolic rate, causing your body to burn up more calories and promoting weight loss.[18] It acts as an anti-inflammatory in the digestive tract,[19] and since 1980, researchers have also demonstrated the benefits of coconut oil on Crohn's Disease and IBS.[20] Its antimicrobial properties also promote intestinal health by killing troublesome microorganisms that may cause chronic inflammation.[21]

What is more, applying coconut oil topically is exceptionally good for keeping your skin young and healthy, as it protects against destructive free-radical formation in the skin cells. Some people have reported success with rubbing the coconut oil on the bottom of their feet to eliminate the hard, dry skin there. Coconut oil can help to keep the skin from developing liver spots and other blemishes caused by aging and overexposure to sunlight,[22] and it also helps to prevent sagging and wrinkling by keeping connective tissues strong and supple.[23] In some cases it even restores damaged or diseased skin.[24]

There is really only one catch with coconut oil—you have to be very careful of the brand and type you choose. From brand to brand, there is a very wide variance in quality due to factors such as the types of coconuts used, the manufacturing process employed to make the oil, and more; these factors will have a major impact on the healthiness and effectiveness of the oil.

Your coconut oil should meet all of these standards:

- Certified organic, USDA standards
- No refining
- No chemicals added
- No bleaching
- No deodorization
- No hydrogenation
- Non-GMO
- From traditional palms only—no hybrid varieties
- From fresh coconuts, not the dried "copra" used in most coconut oils
- Low-level heated only, so it does not damage nutrients

Finally, it is worth mentioning that the excellent health benefits of coconut oil can also be achieved through eating fresh, raw coconuts.

TAKE CONTROL

They're Crazy for Coconut Oil

This coconut oil is awesome. It really makes my veggies come alive with flavor. I also use it on my skin as a body lotion.

—*Elizabeth Thomas* ❧

Fish Oil Is Great Protection For Your Heart

Fish oil contains the omega-3 fats EPA (eicosapentanoic acid) and DHA (docosahexaenoic acid), which are profoundly anti-inflammatory.[25] Fish oil is extremely beneficial for your heart. In fact, it is one of the only nutritional supplements that has an official FDA certification allowing it to claim a beneficial effect on the prevention of heart disease.

Of the many helpful ways that fish oil protects and heals your heart, the following have been found to be especially helpful with fish oil:

- Helps to normalize blood pressure, probably because of its potent anti-inflammatory actions on blood vessel walls, but also because it helps prevent the deposits of plaque and scar tissue from building up and narrowing the walls of your arteries.[26]

- Anti-arrhythmic. It normalizes the rate and rhythm of your heartbeat and helps prevent potentially fatal arrhythmias.[27]

- Anti-thrombotic, meaning that it prevents clot formation and therefore helps protect against strokes and heart attacks. Both of these tragic events can be caused by blood clots.[28]

- Also helps normalize your cholesterol HDL and LDL ratios,[29] bringing the HDL (good cholesterol) up to an optimal range.[30]

Fish Oil Decreases Risk of Cancer

Fish oil offers protection against and treatment of prostate cancer.[31] Tumor growth rates and prostate tumor sizes actually went down in a group of subjects who were given omega-3 fatty acids.

Breast cancer is the second most common cancer in women. Research has shown that fish oil interferes with the progression and metastasis of breast cancer cells.[32] It also seems that fish oil has a preventative effect against colon cancer.[33]

Fish Oil and Your Brain

While fish oil has not been shown to reverse Alzheimer's Disease, it has shown positive benefits for mild cognitive dysfunction induced in rats by beta-amyloid plaque formation, which is the same kind of damage that Alzheimer's Disease causes.[34]

For the rapidly developing nervous system in the unborn, newborns, and children, fish oil is a tremendously helpful supplement to their diet. The expectant mom will find that not only her baby benefits, but fish oil can help her with some of the emotional changes and forgetfulness that may accompany pregnancy and the postpartum period.

TAKE CONTROL

Used Cod Liver Oil in Her 5-Month Physical Rejuvenation

Some time ago, personal issues that had been percolating began to take their toll on me physically, and I suffered an excruciating and severe episode of pancreatitis. I had my gallbladder removed, which landed me in intensive care for two full weeks, only four weeks after my daughter had been born.

I had always prided myself on eating right and exercising, but too many things caught up with me. This year, nine years later (and another daughter added in!), I found myself nearly 60 pounds heavier than I could ever have imagined. I was eating well, or so I thought, compared to most people I knew. But, I wasn't eating the right things.

Late last year, I found this wonderful site called Mercola.com. I had also begun researching more traditional diets and began realizing that much of what I had learned was all wrong. What a shock!

Well, upon reading Dr. Mercola's Take Control of Your Health program, and after implementing his suggestions, including Kefir and Cod Liver Oil, I dove in and within five beautiful months, my previously beautiful body rejuvenated itself!

Thank you, Dr. Mercola! I can once again, even as a 38 year old mother of two daughters, walk down the street and have men—and women—comment on my obviously great health (and looks come back, too!)

—Tambra Warner-Sabatini, Titusville, PA ⍦

Cod Liver Oil in the Winter

One form of fish oil that can be particularly useful in the winter months is cod liver oil. The best way to get vitamin D is from sun exposure. However, if you live in a place that is dark and cold in the winter (as I used to before I started escaping to Maui from the frequently sunless Chicago winters) you will likely become deficient in vitamin D. A high quality cod liver oil is a great choice as a vitamin D supplement, as long as you monitor your blood levels to make sure you do not overdose. Also make sure the cod liver oil is high quality, which means it is free of contaminants and not damaged in the processing.

Cod liver oil has another wonderful benefit, and that is Vitamin A. Vitamin A is abundant in vegetables, but you may not be getting as many vegetables as you really need, especially in winter. The vitamin A in cod liver oil is a tremendous boost to your immune system during the colds and flu season.

Problems with Fish Oil and Cod Liver Oil

There are major problems, however, with contamination of fish. Unfortunately, the world's oceans are so polluted with industrial waste that most commercially available fish have become saturated with many toxins, especially mercury, throughout all the fat and tissues of their bodies.

> The tragedy is that fish used to be one of the healthiest foods on earth, but now you have to be very careful about the type of fish you eat and the source of the fish in order to protect your health.

The majority of electricity in the United States is produced by burning coal, which produces mercury, which finds its way to small waterways and then to the oceans, where it bioaccumulates in the fish. Smaller fish, such as herring, sardines, and anchovies are not so bad, because they have not absorbed as much mercury. The highest concentrations are found in the large carnivorous fish of the ocean: tuna, swordfish, shark, etc. This is because, every stage up, where a bigger fish eats a smaller fish, there is a higher and higher concentration of mercury and other toxins.

In farmed fish, there is not only the problem of mercury, but also PCBs, another poisonous industrial byproduct.

There are a couple of ways around this problem so you don't have to give up this otherwise healthy food. One way is to get distilled fish oil and cod liver oil. Look for a brand that is routinely inspected for the presence of various heavy metals and PCBs. It maintains international standards for purity and quality. Be sure to refrigerate your fish and cod liver oils to slow oxidation.

Great Form of Omega-3—Krill Oil

Another way to get your omega-3 fats is by taking krill oil. Krill are small shrimp or prawn-like creatures, and are small enough that they do not have a chance to accumulate toxins. But krill is a highly concentrated source of the healthy anti-inflammatory omega-3 fats, EPA, and DHA.

Krill are the primary food source of the world's largest animals—the great whales. But krill are not a new source of nutrition for humans and land animals. Krill have been harvested as a food source for both humans and domesticated animals since the 19th century, and perhaps even earlier in Japan, where these small creatures are considered a food delicacy.

> **TAKE CONTROL**
>
> **Fish Oil Very Helpful With PMS**
>
> I find fish oil to be very helpful with PMS problems; I'm sure the heart benefits are there as well. I have had no fishy or other bad after taste and "repeats." It works exceptionally well for me.
>
> —Michelle Gallavan-Orris, Fayetteville, NC ❧

One way in which krill oil is superior to fish oil is that krill oil contains omega-3s in the form of phospholipids, which are little packages that deliver the fatty acids directly to your body's cells. All scientific evidence to date has shown that the safest and most effective carriers of EPA and DHA are these phospholipids. Standard fish oils (and some substandard krill oil brands) lack this phospolipid complex, instead containing omega-3's in the less beneficial form of free triglycerides. This makes the omega-3 fats in krill oil significantly more bioavailable than those in fish oil.

In addition to containing omega-3 fats in phospholipid form, krill oil has another very strong advantage that fish oil does not; krill has high levels of anti-oxidants (more than 47 times the levels found in fish oil). This is especially important for food that contains a high amount of omega-3 fatty acids, because they can turn rancid quite easily in your body and can create free radicals, which are the main culprit in early aging. Krill's combination of anti-oxidants and omega-3 fats is the perfect combination.

Krill also has the advantage of being more digestible than fish oil. Many people have the unpleasant problem of burping up fish oil for a while after they have swallowed it. Krill oil greatly reduces this problem.

One final important factor is that, together with plankton, krill make up the largest biomass on earth. They congregate in dense masses or swarms that can actually turn the ocean's surface pink or red. This makes them one of the most easily renewable food resources available and an excellent nutritional source from an environmental perspective. (Check out Mercola.com for researched and recommended products.)

TAKE CONTROL

No Cramps or Headaches!

I have been taking fish oil for about 10 days now and I already notice a small boost in energy and a better ability to concentrate. But more importantly I didn't experience ANY cramps or headaches that I normally do, due to my menstrual cycle this month. I usually have pretty uncomfortable back pain, cramping and a very severe migraine. NOTHING this month at all! I can't wait to see how I will do after a month or two! (As a side note, I don't get any bad aftertaste or 'belching' later with this product.)

—Allison LeBaron, Tujunga, CA ✎

What About Flax Oil?

Omega-3 fatty acids may also be found in walnuts and flax, so these are beneficial to eat. However, it is important to remember that the fats in these sources are not as effective as the omega-3 fats found in fish oil.

The EPA and DHA acids in fish, cod liver and krill oil have a stronger anti-inflammatory effect than the alpha-linolenic acid or ALA in flax oil. You would have to take about 10–12 times as much flax oil every day to get the same effect. Also, EPA and DHA are the primary omega-3 fats that your body uses. When you take ALA your body needs to convert that fat to EPA and DHA. Those conversions require the enzyme delta-6 desaturase, and this enzyme is typically impaired when high levels of insulin are present.

Since two thirds of us are overweight and others have diabetes, high cholesterol and high blood pressure, this enzyme is inhibited in the vast majority of people and the conversion of ALA to DHA is far less than optimal.[35] In fact using flax instead of fish oil as an omega-3 source has even been shown to increase, not decrease, prostate cancer.[36]

Other Good Fats

Omega-6 fatty acids are to some extent anti-inflammatory, but since most of our foods are already quite high in these, it would not be wise to supplement omega-6 fatty acids.

Omega-9 fatty acids are also healthful. The most common source is olive oil. Remember, however, that you have to be careful not to cook with it at temperatures higher than medium heat. The double-bond at the 9 position easily flips to a trans-configuration and gives you a trans fatty acid. For that reason, I like saturated fats like coconut oil for cooking.

TAKE CONTROL

Lung Condition Clears Up

My cousin recommended mercola.com to me to aid in regaining my health. My illness began with flu-like symptoms, severe cough, loss of weight. In January, I was referred to lung specialist, and began treatment of doxycycline and advair. Symptoms returned within 30 days after treatment stopped. Returned to treatment of doxycycline and advair (steroid) and was informed this could go on for two years. Finished treatment and still felt rotten.

Started Dr. Mercola's Take Control of Your Health Program along with recommended products (probiotic, omega 3 fish oil, and chlorella), along with as much exercise as I could manage. After 30 days, my energy level was greatly increased, and flu symptoms were gone. It is now four months with the Take Control of Your Health Program, and I'm feeling absolutely wonderful. Would recommend to everyone, in fact I do!

—*Susan Skeen, Worland, WY* ⌒

CHAPTER:

Importance of Raw Food

One of the key principles to achieving high-level health is to make sure at least 50 percent of your diet is composed of uncooked (raw) food. To put it simply, this is because there are valuable and sensitive micronutrients in foods, and these are damaged when you heat them.

Cooking foods to any degree (along with processing them) can destroy many of these micronutrients by altering their shape and chemical composition. The end result is a less nutritious and possibly even harmful version of the healthy raw food you started with. While some cooked foods do have their place in a healthy diet, striving to eat mostly raw foods is ideal, and any healthy diet should be composed of at least one-third raw foods.

How It's Possible to Eat All Day and Still Starve

The notion that foods play an enormous role in your health is not new thinking as evidenced by Hippocrates' statement from nearly 2,500 years ago, "Leave your drugs in the chemist's pot if you can heal the patient with food." Unfortunately, this simple statement and smart way of thinking has yet to become a mainstay of American culture.

The concept fell into obscurity by the 19th century. From 1900–1950, marked the discovery of how micronutrient deficiencies such as vitamins and minerals could lead to sickness and disease. This led to "enrichment" of processed foods (adding these vitamins back into the food) to help people regain the health they lost when they replaced whole foods with processed foods.

Today, it is possible to eat all day long and still starve yourself.

Why?

Because if all you eat are junk foods and other foods with little to no nutrition, such as overly cooked foods, you will not receive the nutrients your body needs to function properly, let alone heal disease. All that your body has to run on are the foods you put into it, and it needs the best foods it can get to combat all of the stress and environmental toxins that are virtually impossible to avoid in today's world.

In this way, whole foods certainly can act as "medicine" in that they can protect and heal your body. Another way to look at it is if you fortify your body with healthy nutrients from fresh foods, you likely won't have a need for medicine. Individual foods each have their own unique set of nutrients that meet the varying requirements of your body. This is why it's so important to eat a wide variety of foods—to ensure that your body gets all of the diverse nutrients it needs. Naturally, in order to achieve the most optimal results, you should eat foods as close to their natural state as possible, or in other words, **raw**.

Why Raw Foods Are Better

To get an idea of the healing power of raw foods, consider fresh vegetables, which are among the most nutrient-dense foods. They contain many natural antioxidants including vitamins A, C, E, carotenes, zinc, selenium, bioflavonoids, tocopherols, lutein and quercetin, and many beneficial phytochemicals. These can help to fight age-related and chronic diseases like cancer and heart disease, boost the immune system, fight osteoporosis, lower your risk of diabetes, and slow brain aging. They will also help to alkalinize your system, as most of us are far too acidic.

However, take these same vegetables and cook them, and you will lose a great deal of their nutrients, and therefore their healing capacity. For instance, cooking broccoli in the microwave along with a little water causes it to *lose up to 97 percent* of the beneficial antioxidants it contains. Even steaming it, which is certainly one of the healthier methods of cooking, could cut its antioxidant capacity by 11 percent.[1]

Aside from the nutrients, raw foods contain enzymes, probiotics, and other components that help break down and digest food, balance your body's pH, and perform a huge variety of necessary daily bodily functions. But enzymes are extremely fragile. They're easily deactivated and destroyed through processing and handling and by heat (even at temperatures as low as 72°F—although typically enzyme destruction occurs around 110°F).

So if the only raw food you get is an occasional piece of iceberg lettuce on a sandwich, you simply are not getting enough enzymes, nutrients, and other crucial phytonutrients that your body needs to thrive (you may also find that you have digestive problems, as enzymes and probiotics are key to good digestion).

Can't I Just Take a Supplement?

While you may be tempted to simply pop a few vitamins and assume you're covered nutritionally, eating raw, whole foods will give you more comprehensive nutrition than any multi-vitamin supplement. *This is because the combination of substances in a whole food is more synergistically effective* than a specific dietary nutrient that has been isolated and artificially combined with other nutrients.

A 2004 article published in the *British Medical Journal* demonstrates this concept.[2] The article reviews some of the many benefits of folic acid. Ideally, this nutrient is best obtained through organic, fresh, whole vegetables, but supplement companies (many of these are drug companies) have rushed to provide cheap synthetic lookalikes that simply either do not work or are less effective than the whole food variant that is accompanied with all of its accessory micronutrients that function synergistically to provide the observed benefits.

The form of folate in supplements and in fortified foods is pteroyl-monoglutamate (PGA), a form that does not occur in nature. It is both cheap and stable, unlike most natural forms of the vitamin. The study goes on to warn that we have no idea as to the consequences of using high doses of this cheap synthetic version to reap the benefits of folic acid that researchers have found from natural foods.

Other key reasons NOT to rely on supplements for your nutrition are the many things we *don't yet know* about raw foods, as they contain many yet-to-be discovered beneficial compounds. For instance, according to the Weston A. Price Foundation, butter from cows grazing on fast-growing grasses during the spring contained a compound—known as Activator X—that was more beneficial for bone density and overall health than cod liver oil, but which was not present in the butter at other times of the growing season (and which has yet to be isolated).

Choose Raw Dairy Products, NOT Pasteurized Ones

Only a small percentage of dairy products consumed in America are raw, which is most unfortunate as raw dairy is a health-promoting food. Meanwhile, it's important to look past the National Dairy Council's catchy "Got Milk?" campaign to realize that the milk sold in grocery stores is *not* good for you.

Why?

Because it's pasteurized.

Pasteurization was probably useful when it was first employed in the 1920s to kill germs that were spread during that time due to widespread unsanitary production methods. Today, however, sanitation methods of the dairy industry have greatly improved, making pasteurization unnecessary.

Unfortunately, pasteurization still exists and carries many negative side effects, including:

- Killing beneficial enzymes including phosphatase, which allows the body to absorb calcium from the milk
- Destroying colloidal minerals, which are essential to absorb nutrients the milk would otherwise provide
- Precipitating minerals that cannot be absorbed by the body, contributing to osteoporosis
- Precipitating sugars that cannot be digested and fats that are toxic
- Destroying beneficial bacteria and lactic acids that help to protect your body from disease
- Diminishing the cortisone-like factor in the milk that would otherwise help combat allergies
- Destroying vitamins B12 and B6 in the milk
- Promoting other pathogens in the milk
- Contributing to allergies, osteoporosis, arthritis, heart disease, cancer, tooth decay, colic, disorders of the female reproductive system, and weakened immune systems

Public health officials warn that raw milk poses the risk of transmitting bacteria such as listeria, E. coli, and salmonella, but pasteurizing the milk kills these bacteria while extending the milk's shelf life (which also happens to be more profitable for the dairy industry).

While it is certainly possible to become sick from drinking contaminated raw milk, it is also possible to become sick from almost any food source. But it seems that raw milk has been unfairly singled out as a risk when only a very small risk exists. This excerpt from the Weston A. Price Foundation Web site further states this point:

> Except for a brief hiatus in 1990, raw milk has always been for sale commercially in California, usually in health food stores, although I can remember a period when it was even sold in grocery stores. Millions of people consumed commercial raw milk during that period and although the health department kept an eagle eye open for any possible evidence of harm, not a single incidence was reported. During the same period, there were

many instances of contamination in pasteurized milk, some of which resulted in death.

Why Raw Milk is a Superior Choice to Pasteurized Milk

First and foremost, raw milk is an outstanding source of nutrients, including beneficial bacteria such as lactobacillus acidophilus, vitamins, and enzymes, and it is arguably one of the finest sources of calcium available.

The pasteurization process, which entails heating the milk to a temperature of 150°F for 30 minutes and then reducing the temperature to 55°F, radically changes the structure of the milk proteins (denaturization) and converts the proteins into something far less than healthy. While the process certainly destroys germs and bad bacteria, it also destroys the majority of the milk's beneficial bacteria along with many of its nutritious components.

Then, of course, there is the issue of the antibiotics, pesticides, and growth hormones and the fact that nearly all commercial dairy cows are raised on grains, corn, hay and rendered animals (roadkill, other dead cows, etc.), when in fact, a cow's physiology is designed to eat grass. Milk from grass-fed cows contains beneficial fats like CLA—which has been linked to weight loss and other benefits.

Raw Milk Is Better Than Organic Milk

Although organic milk is certainly far better than non-organic milk because it does not contain harmful pesticide and hormone residues, it is vitally important to understand that raw milk is better than organic milk. Even though it is a challenge to obtain raw milk, it is far better to obtain your milk from raw sources than it is to purchase organic milk.

There simply is no comparison of the quality. Most of the time with organic milk, there is an expensive certification process for the organic label that doesn't add any value to the milk, other than to assure you that the milk was raised under clean conditions. Ideally, you should locate the dairy yourself and do your own inspection. Talk to the farmer and see how the cows are being raised. That beats any type of certification process that can be easily manipulated.

Furthermore, most organic and commercial milk is pasteurized and **pasteurized cow's milk is the number one allergic food in this country.** It has been associated with a number of symptoms and illnesses, including diarrhea, bloating, cramps, skin rashes, colic in infants, arthritis, and acne, just to name a few.

Raw milk, on the other hand, is not associated with any of these problems, and even people who have been allergic to pasteurized milk for many years can typically tolerate and even thrive on raw milk.

As with any food, fresher is always better and this applies to milk as well. Fresh raw milk is creamier and better tasting than pasteurized milk that has a shelf-life of several weeks (ultra-high-temperature milk can be stored without refrigeration for about six months!). Even people who have never liked the taste of milk find that raw milk has a soothing, pleasant taste.

Finding Raw Milk

Obtaining raw milk can be a challenge, though, as it is still illegal in many states, but it is well worth the effort to seek out. In ALL states, farmers can drink unpasteurized milk from their own cows. In fact, there is no law against anyone drinking raw milk, just against selling it in some states.

However, you can purchase raw milk in stores in eight states: California, Arizona, New Mexico, Maine, Pennsylvania, Washington, South Carolina, and Connecticut. Another option is to become a member of a cow-share program, in which you become part owner of a cow, and on a routine basis, pick up your share of raw milk.

You can find out sources of raw milk by going to the Weston A. Price Foundation's "Campaign for Real Milk" Web site, www.realmilk.com, to find a source for raw milk near you.

While you are at it, keep in mind that the ideal raw milk would be from cows that are only fed grass (the exception to this guideline are the cows which live in the north must eat hay during the cold winters when there is no grass). When cows are fed grains, their production of the beneficial fat CLA decreases quite substantially.

The Truth About Raw Eggs

Eggs are a phenomenally inexpensive and incredible source of high-quality nutrients that many of us are deficient in, especially high-quality protein and fat. The yolks are also an excellent food to eat raw.

The first thing you may be thinking is, "But what about salmonella?" The truth is that the risk of contracting salmonella from eggs is actually quite low. A study by the U.S. Department of Agriculture found that of the 69 billion eggs produced annually, only 2.3 million of them are contaminated with salmonella.

The translation is that only one in every 30,000 eggs is contaminated with salmonella. You can even further reduce this risk by following the healthy egg guidelines below.

On top of that, even if you were to get salmonella, if you are healthy, a salmonella infection is not a big deal. You may feel sick and have loose stools, but this infection is easily treated by using high-quality probiotics. You can take a dose every 30 minutes until you start to feel better, and most people improve within a few hours.

The reason eating egg yolks raw is so beneficial is that this preserves many of the highly perishable nutrients they contain, such as lutein and zeaxanthin (which are powerful prevention elements of the most common cause of blindness, age-related macular degeneration).

When eating eggs raw, separate the yolk from the white and only eat the yolk. Raw egg whites contain a glycoprotein called avidin that is very effective at blocking the B-vitamin biotin, and eating them raw could lead to a possible biotin deficiency.

To ensure you are getting the highest quality eggs, here are some important guidelines to follow:

- Only buy eggs that are free-range and organic.

- If you can, buy your eggs direct from a farmer so you can be certain of the quality. In this case, you can leave your eggs at room temperature (no need to refrigerate them).

- If you can't find a farmer, contact the company providing your healthy eggs and find out what they are feeding their chickens. An egg is considered organic if the chicken was only fed organic food. (Meanwhile, if they are using flaxseed to increase the omega-3 fats they won't be as beneficial as if they feed the chickens seaweed or kelp, which have the far more beneficial DHA and EPA.)

- Don't eat the egg if there is a crack in the shell. (If you're not sure, immerse the egg in a pan of cool, salted water. If the egg emits a tiny stream of bubbles, don't eat it, as the shell is porous.)

- Don't eat eggs that have a foul odor, a watery white, or a yolk that's overly runny or breaks easily.

Finally, if you choose not to eat your egg yolks raw, the next best option is to eat them poached or soft-boiled.

Problems With Cooked Foods

Part of the reason why eating foods raw is so beneficial is that you avoid the harmful compounds that are sometimes created when foods are cooked.

For instance, eating egg yolks raw is great, but scramble them and you are oxidizing the cholesterol in the egg yolk, a change that could cause some damage in people with high cholesterol. Cooking foods can also create the following potentially toxic compounds:

- Acrylamide: A cancer-causing chemical byproduct of cooking foods at high temperatures, found in potato chips, French fries, bread, and other foods.

- Heterocyclic Amines (HCAs): Cancer-causing substances formed when meats like beef, pork, and poultry are cooked at high temperatures (such as during charbroiling or barbecuing).

Raw Plant Foods and Dairy, OK, But What About Meat?

Consider the fact that humans are the only animal species that cook their meat—all others eat their meat raw. Eating freshly-killed, raw meat is actually the healthiest way to consume meat as raw meat tends to be free of pathogenic bacteria and contains live enzymes that aid in digestion. Raw meat is commonly consumed in other cultures (think steak tartar, ceviche, and sushi). If you eat raw meat, you should purchase high-quality meat from healthy animals (meaning organic and free-range) as opposed to the antibiotic- and hormone-ridden meat sold in most supermarkets.

However, most people do find this idea hard to stomach. In this case, consuming your meat lightly cooked in water (braising or poaching), at temperatures no higher than 212°F, is preferable to cooking it well-done as it avoids the formation of HCAs.

Organic vs. Grass-fed

If you are seeking alternatives to commercially raised beef a good place to start is Eatwild.com which is the #1 site for grass-fed food facts and sourcing. Beef that is sold in health food grocery markets may say "organic" on the label but if the cows are eating organic corn and hay, there will still be problems inherent with feeding a cow grains.

Also be careful not to be confused by deceptive salesman or farmers. Most all cattle are initially raised on grass but then are shifted to feedlots for the few months prior to their slaughter and are fed large quantities of grain. This is where the damage occurs.

"Grass-fed" used to be a better label to look for but according to grass-fed cattle rancher Lisa Parker, "Some beef labeled as 'grass-fed' is not really grass-fed but that the ranchers wants to sell at a higher price." The following are some examples of beef mislabeled as grass-fed:

1. The calf is raised on grass but then put in a grain feedlot as an adult.

2. The cow is raised mostly on grass but then given high volumes of grain and hay just before slaughter to fatten them up.

3. They may throw a little bit of grass into the feedlots and call it "grass-fed" just to raise the price.

continued

According to Parker, "The legitimate grass-fed ranchers are now looking to use the term 'pasture raised' instead of 'grass-fed' to avoid this abuse but this idea is not uniform as of yet."

The best way to find a source of beef you can trust is to actually meet the rancher personally and ask questions. You can find grass-fed ranchers on Eatwild.com, and there are Amish and Mennonite communities which will sell naturally raised animals. Also note that while cattle can be raised year long on grass in warm southern climates, cattle in the north must eat hay during the cold winter months while the grass is dead.

How to Introduce More Raw Food into Your Diet

The easiest way to begin getting more raw foods in your diet is with vegetables, and specifically vegetable juicing. Juicing vegetables, as described in Chapter Eight, is an incredibly easy way to consume a large amount of vegetables and a large amount of raw food, all at the same time.

It's also easy to make a raw breakfast milkshake using raw eggs, raw milk, and some fruit or raw honey (all according to your nutritional type, of course).

Meanwhile, as you savor the intense flavors of eating fresh, raw foods, you can also savor the time you're saving in the kitchen by not having to cook. Eating raw foods is a great way to save time, and there are plenty of foods that can be eaten raw while on the go. Raw vegetables, raw seeds, raw nuts, and raw dairy all fit into this category—simply tailor your individual choices to fit your nutritional type, and go!

Water Guidelines for a Healthy Body

"Drink more water."

It's a phrase you've probably heard often—from your mother, your doctor or a well-meaning friend—but what you often don't hear is why water is so crucial for your health . . . and that the quality of your water is just as important as the quantity.

But before we delve into the burning question on most everyone's mind when it comes to talking about water (*how much should I drink?*), it helps to understand why getting enough water is so important. Indeed, we can exist without food for months, but without water you can only survive for a few days.

Your body, in fact, is made up mostly of water, which:

- Is essential for digestion, nutrient absorption and elimination
- Aids circulation
- Helps control your body's temperature
- Lubricates and cushions joints
- Keeps the skin healthy
- Helps remove toxins from your body

However, every day you lose water from your body through urine and sweat, and this fluid needs to be replenished. Fortunately, your body has come equipped with a mechanism that tells you when you need to replenish your supply—it's called thirst!

How Much Water Should You Drink?

It seems everywhere you turn, someone is recommending that you drink eight, eight-ounce glasses of water a day. This is the "magic number" commonly believed to prevent dehydration and provide your body with all the fluids it needs. However, this adage may not be as accurate as you have been led to believe.

There is no one universal amount that can accurately predict precisely how much water you should drink. Take, for example, an active high school football player training in the middle of summer and a less active, middle-aged, non-exercising, 100-pound mom during the winter. Clearly they'll have drastically varying water needs.

I used to advise that people follow a more individualized rule of thumb—for every 50 pounds of body weight drink one quart of spring or filtered water per day. This would increase your daily water intake to 12 to 16 glasses for most of us.

However, I soon realized that this was also inappropriate for many people. After much trial and error I have concluded that rather than rely on some formula, individualized or not, it is best to allow your body to dictate how much you should drink. When you use this approach you are able to compensate for the dozens of variables that ultimately contribute to what your daily requirements are.

One way you can achieve this is by observing the color of your urine. Under most circumstances you should strive to have your urine have a very light yellow or straw color. A darker and deeper yellow or even orange may indicate you are dehydrated and not drinking enough water.

The only caveat here is if you are taking riboflavin (vitamin B2) which fluoresces and turns your urine bright yellow you will not be able to peform this test (riboflavin is in most multi-vitamins).

It's also important to sip your water all day long, as opposed to downing a pint of water several times a day. Depending on your size, your body can only process a bit more than a glass of water per hour. If you drink much more than this at one sitting, the extra water will not be used, but rather be flushed down the toilet bowl.

Let Thirst be Your Guide

Meanwhile, your body has an intrinsic sensor—your thirst mechanism—that will give you a nudge when it's time for some water. When your body begins to lose from 1–2 percent of its total water, your thirst mechanism kicks in and tells you, "I'm thirsty, drink some water." If you are healthy, then drinking whenever you feel thirsty should be an adequate guide of how much water you need. You can confirm whether you are drinking enough water by looking at the color of your urine, as mentioned above.

Of course, if you live in a climate that is hot, has high altitude, or low humidity, or you are engaged in exercise or other vigorous activity, you will require more water than normal so be sure to stay well hydrated in these cases. Additionally, as you grow older your thirst mechanism works less efficiently, so if you are elderly, you will want to be sure to drink water regularly, and again make sure the urine is a light, pale yellow color.

Water—Not Soda—Should be Your Beverage of Choice

Clean water is the best beverage to quench your thirst and support your body. If you are currently a soda drinker, one of the easiest and most profound things you can do to improve your health is to trade your soda and other sweetened drinks for water. This would impact a huge number of people, as nearly 50 percent of Americans over the age of four drink soft drinks on any given day.

Meanwhile, most Americans are clueless about health and drink nearly one-fourth of their total daily calories, mostly in the form of soft drinks, sweetened juices and presweetened iced teas.More than one-third of all the added sugars Americans consume come from soft drinks.[1]

High-fructose corn syrup, the sweetener in most sodas, has been linked not only to the obesity epidemic, but it can also harm organs like your liver and pancreas, leading to bone loss, anemia and heart problems, just to name a sampling of its dangers.

Now, here is something startling: in 2005, soft drinks and sweet drinks replaced white bread as the leading source of calories in the average American diet.[2] Aside from obesity (your risk for obesity increases by a whopping 60 percent for each can of soda you drink a day[3]), drinking soft drinks has been linked to:

- Osteoporosis
- Attention deficit disorder (ADD)
- Insomnia
- Kidney stones
- Tooth decay

You clearly have everything to gain from not drinking soda (and certainly not allowing your children to either). That said, the caffeine and sugar in soda can be quite addictive, so you may want to quit "cold turkey" and use the Emotional Freedom Technique (described in Chapter Eleven) to help you make the transition.

Adding a squeeze of lemon or lime juice to your water (if your Nutritional Type allows it) can also give you some of the flavor you may initially miss.

Finally, please remember that even though diet sodas don't contain calories, they contain potentially toxic artificial sweeteners. Switching your regular soda habit to a diet soda one will not help your health in any way (and may actually make it worse), so ditch all the soda (regular and diet) and choose water instead.

Be Wary of Tap Water . . . It Is NOT As Safe As You Think

In an ideal world, you would be able to turn on your kitchen faucet and draw from it a perfectly clean glass of water. In reality, if you are drinking water from your tap you are almost assuredly getting hefty doses of two toxins: chlorine and fluoride.

The irony is that these substances are intentionally added to your tap water under the guise they are killing bacteria or benefiting your health—neither of which is accurate.

Chlorine is added to municipal water supplies to kill disease-causing bacteria in the water itself and in the pipes that transport it. This it does very well because it's a potent disinfectant.

But chlorine also has a dark side. According to the U.S. Centers for Disease Control and Prevention (CDC)[4], chlorine:

- Was used during World War I as a choking (pulmonary) agent (in gas form)

- Is used as a bleach in the manufacture of paper and cloth

- Is used to make pesticides, rubber, and solvents

- Kills harmful bacteria in swimming pool water

- Is used as part of the sanitation process for industrial waste and sewage

From a commonsense standpoint alone, does it make sense to drink something that is capable of poisoning people and killing insects, and which is easily turned into caustic industrial products?

Of course not. When chlorine interacts with organic matter in water, it forms disinfection byproducts (DBPs). Two primary DBP categories are trihalomethanes (TTHMs) and haloacetic acids (HAA5s).

DBPs have been linked to a number of harmful effects, including:

- Cancer in laboratory animals

- Undesirable effects in lab animals' growth and reproduction

- Several studies that have found an increased cancer risk to those using chlorinated drinking water

For instance, six studies that examined a combined total of almost 8,000 people found that men who drank more than two liters of tap water a day ran a 50 percent higher risk of bladder cancer than those who drank half a liter or less.[6]

Other studies also have indicated that drinking chlorinated water could negatively impact human reproduction and development, but the U.S. Environmental Protection Agency (EPA) is holding out on stating conclusively that DBPs cause these health effects, saying more research is needed.

Along with the chlorine, fluoride is also added to U.S. drinking water, and has been for over 50 years in order to prevent dental decay.

Imagine, this drug is being "prescribed" to the entire U.S. population with no consent and no way to track dosage or individual reactions, and without concern for some people's increased vulnerability to the drug. It sounds crazy, but that is exactly what is happening in the United States with water fluoridation.

Not only is the practice unsafe, it is also ineffective for prevention of tooth decay. Data compiled by the World Health Organization shows absolutely no difference in tooth decay in countries that use fluoridated water compared with countries that don't use fluoridated water.[7]

Further, several additional studies have found that tooth decay rates do not increase when water fluoridation is stopped, and in some cases the rates even go down. One U.S. survey, conducted from 1986 to 1987, found that fluoridated water made no difference in tooth decay when measured in terms of DMFT (Decayed, Missing and Filled Teeth), and made a statistically insignificant difference (on about 0.5 percent of 128 tooth surfaces) when measured as DMFS (Decayed, Missing and Filled Teeth Surfaces).[8]

When water fluoridation first began, it was believed that fluoride had to be ingested for it to be effective. However, this has since changed and the dental community now almost unanimously believes that fluoride's benefits result from topical application, not when it is swallowed.

Amazingly in mid–2007 even the American Dental Association, one of the longtime proponents of fluoride, reversed its position on fluoride and did not advise dentists to give babies fluoride because of its adverse effect on bone growth.[9]

Despite fluoride's apparent ineffectiveness, it is still used in the United States, but not without consequence. The fluoride that we

111

ingest from the water supply and from a number of other sources such as toothpaste, mouthwashes, processed food, some vitamin tablets, and beverages like fruit juice, soda and tea is associated with a number of negative health effects. Consider that:

- Fluoride accumulates in your bones, making them brittle and more easily fractured.

- Fluoride accumulates in your pineal gland, which may inhibit the production of the hormone melatonin. Melatonin helps regulate the onset of puberty.

- Fluoride damages tooth enamel (known as dental fluorosis) and may lower fertility rates.

- Fluoride has been found to increase the uptake of aluminum into your brain and lead into blood.

- Fluoride inhibits antibodies from forming in your blood.

- Fluoride confuses the immune system, causing it to attack the tissues in your body. This can increase the growth rate of tumors in people prone to cancer.

Noting these and other health risks and the obvious ethical issue of medicating an entire population without their consent, many European countries have banned water fluoridation.

In the United States, however, nearly all drinking water is fluoridated. This is despite the fact that, in 2005, eleven EPA employee unions called for a moratorium on drinking water fluoridation programs. They further asked EPA management to recognize fluoride as posing a serious cancer risk.[10]

The unions acted in response to an apparent cover-up of evidence from the Harvard School of Dental Medicine connecting fluoridation with a seven-fold increased risk of the fatal bone cancer osteosarcoma. The unions also cited other results similar to those in the Harvard study, and recent work that links the use of silicofluoride fluoridating agents with increased lead levels in water.

Along with chlorine and fluoride in your tap water, other contaminants that sometimes exist in drinking water include:

- Pesticides

- Mercury and arsenic

- Aluminum

- Perchlorate (a primary ingredient in rocket propellant)

- Pharmaceutical and personal care products (PPCPs) including residues of birth control pills, antidepressants, painkillers, shampoos, and many other chemical compounds

While you may be thinking that your water is safe because it tastes, looks and smells fine, please realize that you cannot recognize toxins in your tap water with your senses alone.

Many contaminants are tasteless, odorless and colorless, and others are so harmful that they are measured in "parts per million" or "parts per billion." In other words, just a drop of these poisons added to gallons and gallons of water can be very harmful (but almost impossible to recognize on your own).

This is why I highly recommend filtering your tap water for your optimal health (and not relying on bottled water).

Why I Avoid Using Bottled Water, and Suggest You Do the Same

Many people's first instinct when they hear about the toxins in tap water is to switch over to bottled water. However, bottled water is not the best choice for your clean water needs, and here's why.

In 2004, worldwide consumption of bottled water increased by nearly 60 percent (41 billion gallons). We are on track toward consuming more than 50 billion gallons in 2007. All of this water is pricey, putting a strain on your pocketbook, and, worse, an enormous strain on the environment.

The environmental impact of all those plastic bottles is huge, not only in the massive amounts of resources it takes to make them and transport them around the world, but also in the amount of waste they create.

It takes 1.5 million barrels of oil each year to create enough polyethylene terephthalate plastic to make all of those bottles; that amount of oil could fuel about 100,000 cars for a year![11] In addition, 86 percent of plastic water bottles used in the United States become garbage or litter, and these bottles can take up to 1,000 years to finally biodegrade. Much of this plastic eventually migrates to the ocean and this plastic migration is causing large amounts of the ocean to become plastic garbage heaps and it is destroying enormous quantities of marine life.[12]

Furthermore, drinking bottled water is not even an assurance of purity. In fact, **up to 40 percent of bottled water is tap water** that may be loaded with fluoride.[13] The additional treatment may even be to disinfect the water, which is often done using chlorine. On top of that, it may also be contaminated with the potentially toxic metal antimony.

Among 63 brands of bottled water produced in Europe and Canada, researchers detected concentrations of more than **100 times the typical level of antimony** in clean groundwater (2 parts per trillion). And, after letting bottled water samples sit for six months on a shelf at normal room temperatures, antimony leached from the plastic container into the water and the concentration of antimony exploded by 90 percent among European brands and 19 percent in Canadian brands.[14] These numbers could be even worse if the water was heated as it might be in an attic or garage.

I also recommend avoiding bottled distilled water, unless you are using it therapeutically for a limited time for a specific detox. Though drinking distilled water is sometimes endorsed by natural medicine practitioners, distilled water should be avoided because the physical structure at a molecular level is compromised once it has been distilled. Additionally it has the wrong ionization, pH, polarization and oxidation potentials. Due to the low osmolarity, distilled water can leach the minerals from your body because after distillation it becomes like a vacuum and seeks to replace the minerals it lost by extracting them from your body. Using distilled water for a short term fast or detoxification process might make sense, but you should clearly avoid using it for any extended period of time.

How to Get Clean, Environmentally Friendly Water

Your best option for securing clean, economically priced and environmentally friendly water is to filter your own tap water using a reverse osmosis (RO) filter. RO filters work by squeezing water through a semi-permeable membrane that is tiny enough to keep out contaminants and only let pure water through. RO is also the process used to remove salt from sea water to turn it into drinking water.

It is important to know that the RO filter is only one of three types of filters that are effective at removing fluoride from your tap water. The other two are a water distiller and an Activated Alumina Defluoridation Filter. As mentioned, above, distillation is not your best choice, and the defluoridation filters are far more expensive to use in the long run. For a relatively small investment, RO filters will provide you with clean water for your healthy body, and peace of mind in knowing that the water you and your family are drinking is safe.

As an aside, if you opt for an under-the-sink RO filter, as opposed to a whole-house variety, you may also want to add a filter to your shower to remove chlorine (if you are on your own well, then this is not necessary). As shocking as it sounds, showering in chlorinated water can actually expose you to more of the chemical than drinking it!

CHAPTER:

Planning Your Meals

Once you have made the decision to make nutrition and health a top priority in your life, you must find a way to make it fit with your routine. Admittedly, one of the biggest challenges to eating healthy is finding the time to do so, but anyone and everyone can do it.

If you are healthy, it is easy to take your body for granted. Those who are sick, though, realize just how important their health is. But you don't want to wait until your health goes away to realize that it is one of the most, if not *the* most important aspect of life.

If your car breaks down, you can have it fixed, but if your body breaks down, you can't replace it. Your body needs to last the rest of your life, therefore, it's best to treat it with care. Protect it by being proactive. This includes planning your meals in a healthy way.

Failing to Plan? You're Planning to Fail!

Do you ever get home from work later than expected or find yourself trying to prepare lunch for your kids in the midst of a million other activities? We've all been in these situations, and it's these times when it's most tempting to eat something packaged, processed and a poor choice.

However, you will be amazed that with a little planning you can have a healthy meal ready to eat in about the same time you could stop for fast food, or microwave a nutrition-less convenience food. Here are the top three steps you need to know:

- Once a week, sit down and plan your meals for the week ahead (including snacks). Write them down by day and mealtime, and at the same time start a grocery list of all the foods you'll need to prepare them.

- Make it your goal to find 10–20 healthy recipes that you and your family enjoy. This is all that most families use. It may take some time and trial and error to get to the final ten but it will be well worth the effort.

- Grocery shop once a week, picking up everything you'll need for the following week's meals. This is much more efficient than running out to the store every other day.

Tips for Planning, and Cooking Healthy Meals (Even When Crunched for Time)

To eat healthy, you will need to spend some time in the kitchen. This doesn't mean that cooking and eating will take the place of your full-time job, however, as there are plenty of tricks you can use to create healthy meals even when you're short on time.

Start by making smart choices when you plan your meals for the week. Keep an eye out for foods that can be prepared once but used multiple times throughout the week. For instance, if you cook two chickens on Monday, you'll have plenty left over to use on salads or in a stir-fry later in the week.

Meanwhile, choose recipes that are simple for you to prepare. There's no need to burden yourself learning complex cooking skills (unless you enjoy it and have the time!); simple meals are just as healthy and often the ones your family will love the most. For instance, a big pot of soup or stew can be thrown together relatively quickly, it will satisfy your family, and you can freeze a portion of it for another meal.

Another option would be turkey burgers with a side of quickly cooked greens (or whatever vegetable is appropriate for your nutritional type). This is a quick and easy meal, and if you make a few extra patties you can turn the leftovers into a turkey and vegetable casserole later in the week.

Eating Healthy Even With A Busy Lifestyle

It may be tempting to justify your fast food lunches by saying you "just don't have time to eat healthy," but in the end you are setting yourself up for failure.

Don't let time get the better of you. Once you read through the tips below, you won't be able to make any more excuses; you'll be able to eat nutritious food even if you don't think your schedule allows it.

Cook in Large Batches: Whether you are cooking some grass-fed bison patties or making fermented vegetables like sauerkraut, cooking large batches will assure that you have some left over for the next day.

Almost anything you make can be stored (in glass containers) overnight and eaten as another meal the next day. If you cook even more, you'll also have enough left to freeze for later use.

Leftovers from dinner can even be eaten for breakfast, and in fact, are a healthier choice than the typical American breakfast of cereal, toast, pancakes, bagels, or doughnuts.

Eat a Good Portion of Your Food Raw: As we said in Chapter Five on eating raw foods, there are valuable and sensitive micronutrients that are damaged when you heat foods. Cooking and processing food can destroy these important and valuable micronutrients by altering their shape and chemical composition.

Not only is eating foods raw healthy, it's quick and easy. So when you're planning your meals for the week, remember that every meal doesn't have to be cooked. Plan some raw meals (or raw portions of meals) right into your schedule, taking advantage of tasty and healthy foods like raw vegetables, raw seeds, raw nuts, raw berries, raw dairy, and raw egg yolks.

Prepare Your Lunch the Night Before: It is no mystery that when you are at work, come noontime you will be hungry and looking for lunch. You will have trouble finding high quality, nutrient dense, whole food meals at restaurants and fast-food joints so the key is to think ahead.

Morning can be a very hectic time of day and one way to cut down on things to do in the morning is to make it a habit to prepare your lunch the night before. This will also reduce the risk that you will neglect to prepare a lunch altogether and then decide to pick up some unhealthy junk food later in the day.

It is much easier to eat healthy if you can grab your ready-made lunch from the refrigerator as you head out the door (and remember, leftovers from dinner make a quick and easy lunch or breakfast).

Eat Only When You're Hungry: If it's lunchtime at work and you don't feel hungry, skip it. The worst thing you can do is to go out and grab some fast food and eat it simply because it's time for lunch. Chances are your body can use the break from digestion, and the junk food you would be tempted to get while on the run will only make you tired and sluggish. Occasional fasting is, in fact, a healthy practice for most people. Simply tell yourself you are making a choice to improve your health and live longer.

Be careful not to get carried away with this practice, however, such as skipping breakfast every day. Studies have found that people who skip breakfast are over **four times** as likely to be obese than people who eat something in the morning.[1]

Include the Most Nutritious Foods You Can: When you're looking to save time, one strategy you may use is to combine two things into one, or to "kill two birds with one stone," if you will. This mentality can be applied to many areas of your life and one of them is eating. If you think of food as serving a purpose—to give you the maximum amount of healthy nutrition possible—and then cater your food choices to that purpose, you will save time.

Only eat the most healthy, high-quality foods around and don't waste your time with inferior junk foods.

Know What You're Eating for Dinner Before You Leave Home: If you've planned your meals appropriately, you should know what you're eating for dinner before you leave the house in the morning. This way, you'll know what to take out of the freezer, what to put in the crock-pot, or what to pick up at the market on your way home (in case you've left something out of your weekly trip).

Being organized in this way practically guarantees that you won't panic and give in to fast foods or other unhealthy convenience foods to feed your family.

Choosing Safe Pots and Pans

It is equally as important to choose safe cookware as it is to choose healthy ingredients in your meals. The absolute worst choice for cookware is any type of non-stick pot or pan (such as those coated with Teflon or similar non-stick surfaces).

Non-stick pots and pans are made with perfluorooctanoic acid (PFOA), a dangerous chemical that is thought to cause cancer and birth defects, and which has been found in the blood of more than 95 percent of Americans (PFOA is not only in non-stick cookware, it's also used to make water- and grease-proof products, including microwave popcorn bags and upholstery.)

DuPont, the makers of Teflon, are currently facing a class-action lawsuit for failing to alert customers about Teflon toxicity, and the Environmental Protection Agency (EPA) fined the company millions of dollars for hiding the harmful effects of PFOA and perfluorochemical (PFC) emissions.

The EPA has even called for a Teflon ban; however, it is a voluntary one. So, it's anyone's guess whether these dangerous chemicals will ever be regulated or taken off the market.

The convenience of using non-stick cookware is simply not worth the major risks to your health. You should throw away all of your Teflon-coated pots and pans (so you won't be tempted to use them) and replace them with safe cookware alternatives. These include:

- Enameled Cast Iron Cookware (see Appendix B for more information)

- Ceramic-coated pots and pans

- Stoneware

- Glass

Simple Food Preparation Tips for Your Health

As you get into the swing of your meal planning, you'll find that eating healthy is truly a simple way of life. And here are even more tips to make healthy eating second nature:

- Keep your vegetables fresh. By squeezing as much air out of your vegetable bags as possible (do this by holding the bag against your chest and running your arm over it from bottom to top), you'll double or triple their storage life. (The bag should look like it's vacuum-packed when you're done.)

- If you're using non-organic vegetables, letting them soak in a sink full of water and 4–8 ounces of distilled vinegar for 30 minutes will remove many of the contaminants.

- Another option for cleaning fruits and vegetables if you don't have 30 minutes is to spritz them well with three percent hydrogen peroxide and plain white or apple cider vinegar, then rinse them off under running water (it doesn't matter which spray you use first).

- Keep your kitchen clean using the non-toxic hydrogen peroxide and vinegar duo described above. The paired sprays work exceptionally well in sanitizing counters and other food preparation surfaces, including wood cutting boards.

- When cooking your foods, do so gently. Meat cooked "rare" is preferable to meat cooked "well-done," and foods slow-cooked in crock-pots, steamed, or boiled are preferable to those that are fried, broiled, or barbecued.

- If you need an oil to cook with, coconut oil is an excellent choice because it is nearly a completely saturated fat, which means it is much less susceptible to damage when it is heated (unlike vegetable oils and even olive oil).

- Use herbs and spices liberally in your cooking. Things like parsley, cayenne pepper, oregano, garlic, cinnamon, nutmeg, turmeric, and many others will add bold flavors to your meals, and many are also very healthy.

And there you have it—a practical recipe for planning healthy meals for yourself and your family. Once you get into the habit of this routine, you'll be armed with the ability to whip up nourishing, satisfying, low-maintenance meals for a lifetime.

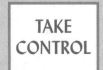

Recovered From Breast and Uterine Cancer

Dr. Mercola's Take Control of Your Health Program was an invaluable help in my fight to recover from both breast and uterine cancer. I only used natural products (except for surgery) and an excellent diet based on Dr. M's cookbook. At this point, three years after diagnosis, I am NED (no evidence of disease). Thank you, thank you!

—*Gisela Tiedemann, Hilton Head Island, SC* ❧

Juicing Your Way to Health

Juicing is an amazing way to accelerate your physical journey to optimal health. However, it is important to understand your nutritional type prior to starting a juicing program. You can find out more information about Nutritional Typing in Chapter Two.

According to Nutritional Typing principles, if you are a carb type, vegetable juicing is STRONGLY recommended. With the patients in our clinic, we strongly encourage it if they expect to regain their health. If you are a mixed type, it is certainly useful to juice; however, protein types need to follow some specific guidelines to make it work for them.

Protein Types and Juicing

If you are a protein type, juicing needs to be done cautiously. The only vegetables that should be juiced are your prime protein type vegetables, which are celery, spinach, asparagus, string beans and cauliflower (including the base).

It is important to keep your serving size of juice to no more than 6 oz., but don't be surprised if you find that as little as 3–4 oz. of juice feels like the right serving size for you. For a protein type, 3–4 oz. of juice is a significant amount.

Also, to make drinking vegetable juice compatible with protein type metabolism (which needs high amounts of fat), it's important to blend a source of raw fat into the juice. Raw cream, raw butter, raw eggs, avocado, coconut butter, or freshly ground flax seed meal are the sources of raw fat that we most recommend. In addition to adding a source of raw fat to your juice, you may also find that adding some or even all of the vegetable pulp into your juice helps to make drinking the juiced vegetables more satisfying to you.

> **TAKE CONTROL**
>
> ### Beating Hepatitis C and Arthritis
>
> I came to see Dr. Mercola for hepatitis C and arthritis. The biggest change that I made was in following the Take Control of Your Health program and eating for my nutritional type. Within a week of making the changes, I noticed a difference in how I felt. I began vegetable juicing and I now drink the juice with every meal. I eat as much organic food as possible along with virtually no sugar or grain. My cravings for sugar and my old way of eating were gone. A great side effect of the program is that I've lost over 35 pounds in two months . . . My arthritis has improved. Since starting the program I can honestly say I've never felt better.
>
> —*Brian McIntyre* ↝

Some Reasons to Juice

There are three main reasons why you will want to consider incorporating vegetable juicing into your health program:

1. **Juicing helps you absorb all the nutrients from the vegetables.** This is important because most of us have impaired digestion as a result of making less-than-optimal food choices over many years. This limits your body's ability to absorb all the nutrients from the vegetables. Juicing will help to "pre-digest"

them for you, so you will receive most of the nutrition rather than having it go down the toilet.

2. **Juicing allows you to consume an optimal amount of vegetables in an efficient manner.** If you are a carb type, you should eat one pound of raw vegetables per 50 pounds of body weight per day. Some people may find eating that many vegetables difficult, but you can easily accomplish it with a quick glass of vegetable juice.

3. **You can add a wider variety of vegetables in your diet.** Many people eat the same vegetable salads everyday. This violates the principle of regular food rotation and increases your chance of developing an allergy to a certain food. But with juicing, you can experience a wide variety of vegetables that you may not normally eat.

If you are new to juicing, I recommend a mid-priced juicer. The cheap centrifugal juicers (like the Juiceman) break easily, produce low quality juice and are very loud, which may contribute to hearing loss. My favorite juicer is the Omega Juicer.

Many of my patients thought that juicing would be a real chore, but the majority were pleasantly surprised to find that it was much easier than they thought it would be. This is partly related to the fact that you should only start by juicing vegetables that you enjoy eating non-juiced. The juice should taste pleasant—not make you nauseous.

It is important to listen to your body when juicing. Your stomach should be happy all morning long. If it is churning or growling or generally making its presence known, you probably juiced something you should not be eating. Personally, I've noticed that I can't juice large amounts of cabbage, but if I spread it out, I do fine.

Lesson 1: Drink vegetable juice for breakfast.

Vegetable juice is a great breakfast when balanced with some essential oils and a bit of chlorella. Please remember that vegetable juice and fruit juices are two completely different substances in terms of nutrition. Ideally, you should avoid fruit juices. Although vegetable juice is processed, it doesn't raise insulin levels like fruit juice. The only exceptions would be carrot and beet juice (and most vegetables that grow underground), which function similarly to fruit juice.

Lesson 2: Get ready to juice!

Step 1: Now that you're ready for the benefits of vegetable juice, you need to know what to juice. I recommend starting out with these vegetables, as they are the easiest to digest:

- Celery
- Fennel (anise)
- Cucumbers

These aren't as nutrient dense as the dark green vegetables, which should be avoided if you are a protein type with exception of spinach, Once you get used to these initial three vegetables, you can start adding the more nutritionally valuable, but less palatable, vegetables into your juice.

Vegetables to avoid include carrots and beets. Most people who juice usually use carrots. The reason they taste so good is that they are full of sugar. I would definitely avoid all vegetables that grow underground to avoid an increase in your insulin levels.

If you are healthy, you can add about one pound of carrots or beets per week. I do believe that the deep, intense colors of these foods provide additional benefits for many that are just not available in the green vegetables listed above.

Step 2: When you've acclimatized yourself to juicing, you can start adding these vegetables:

- Red leaf lettuce
- Green Leaf lettuce
- Romaine lettuce

- Endive

- Escarole

- Spinach

Step 3: After you're used to these, go to the next step:

- Cabbage

- Chinese Cabbage

- Bok Choy

An interesting side note: cabbage juice is one of the most healing nutrients for ulcer repair, as it is a huge source of vitamin U.

Step 4: When you're ready, move on to adding herbs to your juicing. Herbs also make wonderful combinations, and there are two that work exceptionally well:

- Parsley

- Cilantro

You need to be cautious with cilantro, as many cannot tolerate it well. If you are new to juicing, hold off. These are more challenging vegetables to consume, but they are highly beneficial.

Step 5: The last step is to use just one or two of these leaves, as they are bitter:

- Kale

- Collard Greens

- Dandelion Greens

- Mustard Greens (bitter)

When purchasing collard greens, find a store that sells the leaves still attached to the main stalk. If they are cut off, the vegetable rapidly loses many of its valuable nutrients.

> One important note: I prefer to juice my vegetables at room temperature. I leave my vegetables out overnight, or for at least one hour in the morning, as I do not enjoy drinking cold fluids, especially when it is cold outside.

Lesson 3: Make your juice a balanced meal.

Balance your juice with protein and fat. Vegetable juice does not have much protein or fat, so it's very important for you to include these fat and protein sources with your meal.

- **Use eggs.** Eggs will add a significant amount of beneficial fats and protein to your meal. An egg has about 8 grams of protein, so you can add two to four eggs per meal. I suggest that you blend the whole eggs raw, right into the vegetable juice. The reason I advocate this is because once you heat the eggs, many of their nutrients become damaged. If you are concerned about salmonella, purchase organic eggs; it's unlikely you'll have any problems.

  There is a potential problem with using the entire raw egg if you are pregnant. Biotin deficiency, a common concern in pregnancy, could be worsened by consuming whole raw eggs.

  > Please read my recent article, "Raw Eggs for Your Health—Major Update" on the website for further information on consuming raw eggs.

- **For increased satiety, blend in some seeds**. If you get hungry easily after juicing, put your juice and seeds in the blender to make a higher fat drink. Seeds are full of protein and essential fatty acids that bring a juice into balance beautifully. I recommend pumpkin and flax seeds. If you use flax seeds use a coffee grinder to grind them first and drink immediately after blending into the juice.

- **Use chlorella.** Chlorella is an incredibly powerful nutrient from the sea and is a form of algae. I use it quite a bit for mercury detoxification, as it binds strongly to mercury to eliminate it from the body. The normal dose is one teaspoon in the juice. However, about 30 percent of people cannot tolerate the chlorella. If it makes you nauseous, you should definitely avoid it. The advantages of chlorella are:

    —Provides a high source of chlorophyll
    —Adds magnesium and protein
    —Binds to heavy metals and pesticides to promote their removal from the body

If you have high iron or vitamin D levels, you will want to avoid chlorella, as it is loaded with both of these nutrients.

- **Add spirulina.** Spirulina is another algae that has many similar benefits and is a good balance to chlorella. However, it does not bind to heavy metals like chlorella.

- **Consider a protein powder.** I personally prefer to drink raw eggs for my breakfast protein. Fresh juice mixed with a protein powder is also a very convenient meal. Whey protein is the best type of powder as it is the most complete protein and the easiest to digest. Although whey protein is from milk and many people have lactose intolerance or an allergy to dairy, the major protein in milk that causes an allergy is casein. Fortunately, whey protein does not contain casein. So most people digest whey protein quite well. The most popular protein powders are the made from soy protein, which I do not recommend due to negative effects unfermented soy has on the body.

- **Add some garlic.** I like to add one clove of garlic in my juice, as it incorporates the incredible healing potential of fresh garlic. I strongly advise you to do this regularly to balance out your bowel flora. The ideal dose is just below the social threshold where people start to notice that you have eaten garlic. One large clove, two medium cloves, or three small cloves is the recommended dose.

- **Add oil.** But not just any oil! I highly recommend cod liver oil for the winter months and fish oil for the summer months. However, if you live in a primarily sunny climate, I wouldn't advise taking cod liver oil. The reason for this is that cod liver oil has a level of vitamin D that can be toxic to those in very sunny climates. The dose for cod liver oil or fish oil is one teaspoon for every 25 to 40 pounds of body weight. Please note that cod liver oil can raise your vitamin D levels to unhealthy ranges. Ideally, you should have your doctor monitor your vitamin D levels with a blood test while taking cod liver oil.

The reason why adding oil (fat) to your vegetable juice may be helpful is that fat can help you better absorb the vitamin K from your vegetable juice as *vitamin K* is a fat soluble vitamin. Vitamin K is very important for gluing the calcium into your bone matrix and helping you build stronger bones. Additionally, new research suggests that vitamin K significantly reduces calcification in the arteries. Adding raw egg yolks, as described above, will also help you to absorb all the vitamin K from the juice. You could also use flax as a source of omega-3 fat, but many people have problems digesting it.

Lesson 4: Make your juice taste great.

If you would like to make your juice more palatable, especially in the beginning, you can add these elements:

- **Coconut:** This is one of my favorites! You can purchase the whole coconut or use unsweetened shredded coconut. It adds a delightful flavor and is an excellent source of fat to balance the meal. Coconut has medium chain triglycerides, which have many health benefits.
- **Cranberries:** You can also add some cranberries if you enjoy them. Researchers have discovered that cranberries have five

times the antioxidant content of broccoli, which means they may protect against cancer, stroke, and heart disease. In addition, they are full of phytonutrients and can help women avoid urinary tract infections. Limit the cranberries to about 4 ounces per pint of juice.

- **Lemons:** You can also add half a lemon (leaving much of the white rind on). If you are a protein nutritional type, you will not want to use lemons, as they will push your pH in the wrong direction.

- **Fresh ginger:** This is an excellent addition if you can tolerate it. It gives your juice a little "kick"!

Lesson 5: Drink your vegetable juice right away or store it very carefully.

Juicing is a time-consuming process, so you'll probably be thinking to yourself, "I wonder if I can juice first thing and then drink it later?" This isn't a great idea. Vegetable juice is perishable, so it's best to drink all of your juice immediately. However, if you're careful, you can store your juice for up to 24 hours with only moderate nutritional decline.

To store your juice:

1. Put the juice in a glass jar with an airtight lid and fill it to the very top. There should be a minimum amount of air in the jar, as the oxygen in air (air is about 20 percent oxygen) will "oxidize" and damage the juice. You can also use a "Food Saver" (See TakeControlofYourHealth.com) if the juice is stored in a ball jar, to evacuate the air from the container. This is not necessary if the jar is completely filled with fluid but recommended if it is partially filled.

2. Wrap the jar with aluminum foil to block out all light. Light damages the juice.

3. Store it in the refrigerator until about 30 minutes prior to drinking, as vegetable juice should be consumed at room temperature.

Most people juice in the morning, but if that does not work out well for your schedule, please feel free to choose whatever mealtime works out best for your lifestyle.

Lesson 6: Clean your juicer properly.

We all know that if a juicer takes longer than 10 minutes to clean, we'll find excuses not to juice at all. I find that using an old tooth-brush works well to clean any metal grater. For the Omega, the whole process takes about 5 minutes. Whatever you do, you need to clean your juicer immediately after you juice to prevent any remnants from contaminating the juicer with mold growth.

WARNING: Don't follow the juicing recommendations that come with the juicer, as they most often emphasize the high sugar carrot and fruit combinations.

TAKE CONTROL

Juicing Helped Elizabeth Conquer Osteoporosis at 60

Here's a story from Elizabeth, one of our Optimal Wellness Center patients:

"As a woman approaching 60 years of age, I knew I didn't want to go the usual route of taking medicines for my recently diagnosed osteoporosis. Because I knew from past experience that taking potent drugs often left me feeling worse instead of better, I decided to take a more nontraditional approach to my healthcare and seek out the services of a holistic doctor.

I launched a search for holistic practitioners via the internet, and it was there that I found Dr. Mercola's Optimal Wellness Center and the wealth of information contained in his website, mercola.com.

On mercola.com, I read helpful article after helpful article until I was convinced that Dr. Mercola had the information and resources

I needed to fight the debilitating disease that I knew osteoporosis could become. I became a patient of the Optimal Wellness Center, and after receiving a thorough examination and evaluation, using several diagnostic tests and procedures, Dr. Mercola and his staff were able to determine a course of action that would put me on the road to better health.

Following their recommendations, I was gradually able to eliminate grains from my diet, drink plenty of fresh green vegetable juices daily and eat those foods that an administered nutritional type test indicated would most benefit my health. With my copy of "Dr. Mercola's Take Control of Your Health Program," in hand, I was well on my way to discovering delicious grain-free recipes (and I even invented a few of my own) to help me eat right for my nutritional type.

I was able to incorporate many other recommendations and lifestyle changes into my daily living. These included, among other things, drinking plenty of good quality water daily, weight training at the local fitness center, practicing methods of relaxation and utilizing a technique called EFT (Emotional Freedom Technique) for the relief of physical as well as emotional pain. After two years, I returned to my local hospital to repeat the bone density scan that had revealed my osteoporosis just two years prior. I was elated to find that not only had I stopped losing bone mass, but there was evidence that my bone mass had actually increased.

I was so relieved to know that my efforts had paid off and that by taking charge of my own health, I had found Dr. Mercola. I was glad, also, that I had made the necessary changes to my lifestyle that put me on the road to better health." ❧

Take Control of Your Exercise Plan

This chapter was written with the help of Ryan Lee and Tony Bruno, both expert personal trainers, and Dr. Al Sears, a prominent physician specializing in exercise therapy.

First, let's start by dispelling many of the common exercise myths and give you some simple, straightforward fitness plans so you can get started right away and get into top shape.

What's Your Reason to Exercise?

Before you begin any exercise program, you must first answer the reason why. Why do you want to exercise? What has driven you to purchase this book and more specifically, to read this chapter?

Maybe it's simply because you want to look better on the beach. Or your doctor said you must begin to exercise. Perhaps you want more energy to play with your children. Maybe you are tired of buying bigger pants sizes each year and want to regain control of your weight and your health.

It's not enough to just say "I want to exercise." You need a strong reason if you want to have any chance of succeeding, and you really have to commit to it. It's not always easy to stick to an exercise plan, especially when it's so much easier to watch TV or just read on the couch. When you have a strong incentive to exercise, everything else will fall into place.

And with the easy-to-follow workout plans here, it's easy to take control of your exercise!

The Aerobic Training Myth

My introduction to exercise was with Dr. Ken Cooper's 1968 book: *Aerobics*, which taught that the best way to get fit is long-distance running. Even though it was not one of my favorite things to do, for the past 38 years I have regularly exercised. For the past 15 years it has been 45 minutes, three times a week. Up until 2006, I have lectured my patients and newsletter readers that if they want to lose weight, they should do 45–60 minutes of intense aerobic exercise (like running) every day.

In 2005 I offered a cruise for Mercola.com newsletter subscribers to join me on a fun vacation and learn more about their health. Over dinner, one of the cruise guests asked both myself and my co-author, Dr. Kendra Pearsall, what we recommended in terms of exercise to lose weight. I told her to run 45–60 minutes every day. None of the people in attendance seemed very excited about that prospect.

To my shock and irritation, Dr. Pearsall offered a different opinion and said, "The research I've read shows that high-intensity anaerobic exercise such as weight lifting has far greater benefits for weight loss than aerobic exercise. In fact, 20–30 minutes of aerobic exercise **per week** is all you really need in conjunction with a weight training regimen of three times a week." Dr. Pearsall was very influential in helping me seek additional insights on this issue and eventually I realized she was right (why do women always have to be right?). In fact, Dr. Pearsall and I have created an online weight loss program (ENLITA.com) based on cutting edge research and natural lifestyle changes.

I am entering nearly my fourth decade of running, but in the last five years or so it has become crystal clear that this simply is not the best way to achieve comprehensive fitness. Although I still believe that aerobic training is part of a good overall program, it simply cannot be your exclusive form of exercise. This is good news as it means you can get fit in LESS time.

I now believe that a combination of aerobic, high-intensity and strength training are more appropriate. Ideally it would be best to combine this with some sport that you can regularly participate in. I happen to enjoy tennis and play singles whenever my schedule allows. I find this far more enjoyable than long distance running.

Ryan Lee shared with us his story about how he discovered that exclusive aerobic exercise was NOT the best way to get in shape:

> My view began to change when I started to pay attention to other athletes. You see, I ran competitive track and field in college and I was a sprinter. In essence, I never really ran more than 200 meters at a time (the length of 2 football fields).
>
> My fellow sprinters and I all trained doing anaerobic exercise the same way: short bursts of speed and zero distance running. We worked out at a very high intensity and took some rest to recover before we sprinted again. We never did distance running—just sprints with rest (called interval training) and in practice we rarely ran more than 150 meters at a time.
>
> And all the 'distance' runners trained the same way: they ran mile upon mile upon mile. No rest, just long slow aerobic training.
>
> So here was the interesting thing . . . all of my fellow sprinters and myself, looked really lean, muscular, and athletic. We all had a low body fat percentage and had the type of physique most people aim for.
>
> It took me many years to realize that the distance runners looked very different from sprinters. They had a rail-thin appearance. Even their faces had a drawn look. They looked older and 'softer' with low muscle tone. In other words, they just didn't look healthy.

The Problem With Aerobics

Here's the biggest problem with aerobic training: your body is quite good at adaptation.

Your body is very adept at trying to help you in your times of need. If you don't eat, your body will slow down your metabolism so you don't starve to death. And if you're thirsty, your body will retain more water.

The same holds true for aerobic exercise. The more aerobic training you do, the more efficient you get at it.

I know what you're thinking: isn't it good for your body to get more efficient at it? Efficiency is good up to a point . . . but if you persist with aerobic training, your body's adaptation may actually do more harm than good.

For example, as a beginner you may only be able to run one mile, after a while, the one mile will become easier and now you must run two miles to get the same benefit. So you will keep going longer and further and the cycle really never ends.

It's the same with aerobics classes. When you do your first one-hour class it might be difficult. But after a few classes it becomes easier. After awhile, you might need to do two classes to get the same benefit you had from just one class.

Did you ever notice there are a lot of overweight aerobics instructors out here? The instructor teaches the class repeatedly, his or her body gets used to the volume/intensity, and over time the class does not create enough demand on the metabolism to burn fat. Exercise scientists call this phenomenon "chunky aerobic instructor syndrome."

The basic point is that you can not do the same workout over and over and expect different results! You must continually change the exercise variables such as duration, frequency, and most importantly, intensity.

Train, Don't Drain

On the other hand, we're not saying you have to become a full-time sprinter or spend an hour every day lifting weights.

Contrary to popular belief, most professional athletes do not spend hours in the gym. Professional strength and conditioning coaches give their athletes time-efficient workouts, and their number one goal is to keep them healthy! Renowned fitness expert, Paul Chek has said, "Train, Don't Drain." Working out harder and longer is not the answer and personal trainers like Ryan Lee and Tony Bruno, who are in the trenches with clients every day, couldn't agree more with Paul.

The less time athletes are in the gym and the more time on the field or court practicing their sports skills, the better. In other words, do your workout as quickly and efficiently as possible—then get back to living!

EPOC is the Key

EPOC stands for Excess Post-Exercise Oxygen Consumption. It's the oxygen your body consumes when you are done exercising. If you do aerobic training, nothing much happens after you are finished with your workout.

But when you do high intensity (anaerobic) training, you have an increased rate of oxygen intake for a long time afterwards. A recent study shows increased oxygen consumption of up to 38 hours AFTER your workout.

That's why high intensity-type training is so valuable. *It's what happens after you stop training that gives you the benefit.*

Again, there is no proof of an increased EPOC for aerobic training, but there is a tremendous benefit for high intensity anaerobic training as **it will help change your body's thermostat for burning calories at all times, even when you are sleeping.**

The Fat Burning Zone Lie

The traditional exercise advice states that to burn the most fat during your exercise, you should do aerobic exercise at 60-80% of your maximum heart rate.

I have to tell you that's one of the biggest myths in fitness. Here's the truth:

The amount of calories and fat burned per unit of exercise is not really a factor! You need to start thinking a much bigger picture than fat and calories burned, as there are far more issues involved. An exercise program using high-intensity anaerobic exercise affects your enzymes, mitochondria, blood sugar, insulin, leptin, and other hormones, protein synthesis, brain activity, and many other factors greater than simple calories burned. It is these other factors that will reset your thermostat to **burn calories while you are not exercising**, which is the far more important issue.

I've included two exercise plans for you to follow, one by Dr. Al Sears and the other by Ryan Lee. They are both excellent. You might try them both and use the one that seems to work best for you, or you might wind up doing each of them at different times.

Take Control Of Your PACE™ And Transform Your Fat Into Muscle

Nature did not program you to stay fit with the traditional methods you've been told. Long duration exercise programs confuse your body into starving muscle and storing fat. But if you exercise in brief bursts, in only a few minutes a day, you can signal your body to rebuild its strength and convince it you don't need the stored fat. You then regain the muscular and lean physique that is your true heritage.

Dr. Sears created a program called PACE™, that stands for Progressively Accelerating Cardiopulmonary Exertion. You will find it's unlike any program you've ever used. It's fast, it's fun, and . . . it actually works. And one of the best benefits of the program is that you are able to achieve phenomenal levels of fitness with far less time than you would in a typical aerobics program.

Progressivity: Progressivity is simply advancing your exertion over time, week by week. What makes all exercise effective is that little bit extra you do this week that you didn't do last week. Start off easy and gradually add resistance or pick up the pace.

Acceleration: At first, it will take you longer to get your breathing and heart rate up. But as you get more accustomed to the challenge, you will gear up faster. As your conditioning increases, you *accelerate* your adaptive response by pushing yourself a little sooner or quicker in your program. This trains your body to adapt to demand quicker.

Use briefer and briefer episodes of gradually increasing intensity.

Cardiopulmonary Exertion: This simply means choosing an activity that will give your heart and lungs a bit of a challenge for your PACE™ program. What you will use will depend on your level of fitness. The important thing, again, is that the challenge advances gradually through time.

Sample PACE™ Progression Plan

Week 1 & 2: First, choose an activity that you are able to change pace at, and measure it. Running, cycling, climbing stairs, working on an elliptical trainer, or even walking are all good activities. Start with 20 minutes at a comfortable pace every other day. If you can't make 20 minutes of continuous activity, take rests as needed. See how much you can comfortably vary the pace. Observe how it makes you feel afterwards. Better yet, keep a log to record your changes in exertion.

Week 3 & 4: Focus on gradually and gently increasing your pace and intensity of your 20-minute workout. Record your progress.

Week 5 & 6: Now break those 20 minutes into shorter intervals. Two eight-minute bouts of exercise with 4 minutes of rest in between will work at first. Now it will be easier to increase intensity of those shorter bouts.

Week 7 & 8: Focus on gradually decreasing the time it takes you to reach your point of highest intensity. This is the principle of acceleration. You are conditioning yourself to respond faster next time. Your intervals will get shorter as your body's speed of adaptation improves. Continue on this cycle.

Beyond Week 9: Rest for 1 week. Now for the fun part. Your body has regained its natural rapid response capability. Gradually break your 20 minute interval every other day into shorter mini-intervals. Try 3 five minutes intervals with 2 three minute rests between. With practice you will change these to 4, then 3, then 2, or even 1 minute intervals of gradually progressing intensity.

If you succeed in achieving the level of fitness for very brief but maximally intense episodes you will find that even 30 seconds is a long time for 100 % effort. **My favorite**: 2 minute warm up, then 8 one minute cycles with one minute rest intervals between.

TAKE CONTROL

Commitment to Exercise And A New Way of Life

I first came to know about Dr. Mercola when I saw him on TV. From there, I subscribed to the newsletter and purchased Take Control of Your Health Program which has been extremely helpful to me.

I have finally made a commitment to a new way of life. I have changed how I eat and am very aware of what I do on a daily basis and how it impacts my health. The most important thing is I am finally committed to exercising 5 days a week no matter what. I can hardly believe how much better I feel!

Thank you Dr. Mercola for all the work you do on your newsletter. Sincerely,

—*Brenda Merrick, Flat Rock, IL* ↦

To learn more about the PACE program visit:
Mercola-pace.com/

Here's an example of a favorite beginning exercise: swimming. Swimming has very little risk of injury:

Note: You will need a waterproof watch or keep a stopwatch on the edge of the pool. You can keep it running, and glance at it to note your time.

Swimming with PACE™

Week	Exercise Minutes	Rest Minutes	Intensity Level
1 & 2	20	0	3
3 & 4	8		3
		4	
	8		4
5 & 6	4		4
		4	
	4		6
		4	
	4		5
7 & 8	4		4
		3	
	3		6
		3	
	2		7
		2	
	3		5

After 8 weeks, stop. Rest for a week and repeat the cycle with something new added. Change your cycle of breathing, throw in a new stroke, or use swimming fins for added resistance. You can repeat these cycles many times as long as you are adding something new to each cycle. After 2 or 3 eight-week cycles I usually switch to a different form of PACE exercise. Bicycling and swimming make excellent alternating PACE cycles. Remember, changing demand mimics the natural environment.

You can find many more variations of PACE programs directly from Dr. Sears on our resource page at TakeControl-ofYourHealth.com

Sample Workouts and Progressions By Ryan Lee

Sample Sprinter Workout Progression

Here's a simple program to follow. You can do this on a cycle, running on a track, or even jumping rope.

1. Sprint for 15 seconds (beginning exercisers should slowly work up to sprinting with slow jogging or fast walking).
2. Rest for 30-45 seconds.
3. Repeat for a total of 10 minutes.
4. Add 2 more minutes every week until you get to 20 minutes.

Sample Quatro Fitness Workout

When I am time-crunched, I like to do my Quatro fitness workouts. Each workout takes just 4 minutes, and they are easy to remember. There's no need for complex math equations and no need to remember hundreds of exercises. In fact, you can get quite fit with just 3 or 4 different exercises.

Each four minute round consists of **eight sets**. A complete set lasts for exactly 30 total seconds (includes work and rest). When you total up the eight sets of 30 seconds, it comes to 4 minutes. It's that simple.

When you become more fit, you can **work up to 3 total rounds**—which would equal 12 minutes of exercise. You can even spread the workouts throughout the day.

Here's the most basic example of what one complete four-minute round would look like using just 4 different exercises. This workout would work every muscle in your body.

Sample 4-Minute Round

Do as many repetitions of each exercise as you can in each set with good form.

Set #1: Push-ups (20 seconds)
Rest #1 (10 seconds)

Set #2: Bodyweight Squats (20 seconds)
Rest #1 (10 seconds)

Set #3: Pull-ups (20 seconds)
Rest #1 (10 seconds)

Set #4: Stability Ball Crunch (20 seconds)
Rest #1 (10 seconds)

Set #5: Push-ups (20 seconds)
Rest #1 (10 seconds)

Set #6: Bodyweight Squat (20 seconds)
Rest #1 (10 seconds)

Set #7: Pull-ups (20 seconds)
Rest #1 (10 seconds)

Set #8: Stability ball crunch (20 seconds)
Rest #1 (10 seconds)

Sample Strength/Sprint Combos

Here's another fun and challenging workout. I like to perform this one on the track.

—Sprint 100 meters (the straightaway)

—Perform 10 pushups

—Walk 100 meters (the turn)

—Perform 10 bodyweight squats

—Sprint 100 meters (the straightaway)

—Perform 15 crunches

—Walk 100 meters (the turn)

Repeat the workout for a total of 4 laps.

Progression tips:

> Add more repetitions to each exercise
>
> Walk faster during the rest
>
> Add a lap onto the workout

More Workouts:

These workouts are just the tip of the iceberg.

If you'd like more workout ideas, visit takecontrol ofyourhealth.com/exercise. Have access to over 100 different websites, each one filled with sample workouts. Or visit Mercola.com/RyanLee

Taking Responsibility Will Increase Your Chances of Success

One of the key components to exercise success is taking complete responsibility. That's correct - your success is up to you. If you miss a day or a week or a month, don't blame anyone else but yourself. Don't blame your spouse, your children, or your job—you must accept 100% responsibility.

This is actually a very healthy approach to take for nearly every aspect of your life. So many of us have the tendency to quickly place the blame for whatever is wrong in our life on our circumstances or others. While this is typically a very convenient approach, it is not a very empowering one.

A simple and powerful illustration when you are tempted to blame someone or something else for your problems is to point your hand at whatever you believe the problem to be. If you look at your hand you will see your forefinger pointing forward, but if you notice your last three fingers, they will be pointing directly back towards you. This is a terrific illustration that demonstrates that most of the time when you are blaming others, it really is your responsibility, not theirs.

If your circumstances or someone else is responsible for your state or condition, then it gives you much less power and freedom to change your situation. Many are reluctant to take full responsibility for not succeeding in their life, but doing so is one of the most powerful choices you can make.

When you take responsibility for everything in your life, only then can you truly take control. This is true not only for exercise and health, but your happiness, your job, your marriage, and your money.

It might have been easy to make excuses about exercising. Excuses like "I don't have enough time" or "I can't afford a personal trainer". But those days are now officially over.

Right now I am going to show you how to get fit in less time than you ever imagined.

Take responsibility and from this day on—no more excuses!

Even Rocket Scientists Benefit from Exercise

TAKE CONTROL

Roy Thatcher from Tucson, AZ wrote in to tell me about his story and how he benefitted from exercise and healthy eating:

I have a Ph.D. in Particle Physics from a top university and was head of a small department at the nation's top High Energy Physics Lab when I had a stroke that ended my career and could easily have ended my life. The stroke ended my career at the Lab and I was struggling with severe memory deficits that made it next to impossible to remember anyone's name. I could walk but had a very severe limp.

I worked incredibly hard with good professional help to get my mind, and in particular, my memory to work properly. I made progress, but it was very slow and got slower until 12 months after the stroke, I was making no discernable progress any longer. At this point I was feeling really desperate because I had developed bladder cancer as well.

Shortly after this, I found Dr. Mercola's web site and began subscribing. At first I was very skeptical but I began to follow his suggestions. I began to feel better and better. I joined a health club. I whipped the bladder cancer and I think my greatly improved diet played a real role in beating the cancer and getting back into shape.

Soon I was doing yoga 2 to 3 times a week and began to square dance and ballroom dance at least once a week. My memory for names is coming back. I still do not have the memory for names that I had before the stroke, but it now as good as many of my friends of about the same age (and it is steadily getting better). I bought Dr. Mercola's book, Take Control of Your Health, as soon as it became available.

I have brought my weight down from 190 to 175 pounds, work out regularly and am eating better than I ever have. It is amazing that I feel so good and can do so much. Dr. Mercola, thank you more than I can express. ॐ

Exercise is a critical component of good health, especially as you age. Exercise will help you:

- *Sleep better*

- *Lose weight, gain weight, or maintain weight, depending on your needs*

- *Improve your resistance to fight infections*

- *Lower your risk of cancer, heart disease and diabetes*

- *Help your brain work better, making you smarter.*

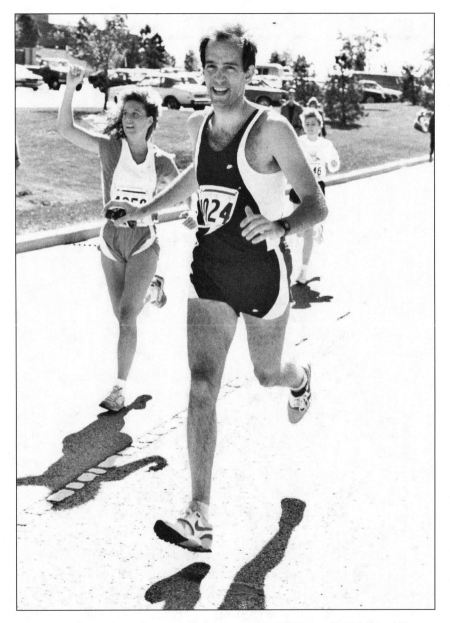

Me and my sister Janet running a major 10K run in 1987. (She placed second in her age category and I was pacing her.)

CHAPTER:

IO

Sunlight and Health

For decades now, the media and nearly every health care "expert" has warned you that the sun is dangerous. At best, you have been told, it will wrinkle your skin and age you prematurely. At worst—and it is a very grim worst case scenario indeed—you have been told that it will greatly accelerate your risk of cancer. You have been told that on a sunny day, you need to slather yourself with sunblock, or a dire fate awaits you.

Doctors, health officials, advertisements commercials, beauty experts, corporations, and well-meaning friends all herald the same message: the sun is your enemy. Too much sun can kill you. You need to stay out of the sun to be safe.

The only problem is, it's all been a distortion of the truth.

That's not to say that sunlight can't be harmful. Of course it can be; the sun is a powerful source of energy and needs to be respected. Anyone who has ever gotten a sunburn knows that sunlight, in large enough quantities, most certainly can damage your skin.

But the fact is that anything, no matter how healthy, can be harmful to you if you receive or consume excessive amounts not consistent with health, and sunlight is no exception. But there is little scientific evidence to justify the massive public health campaigns that recommend avoidance of the sun.

Not Getting Sun Exposure INCREASES Your Risk of Cancer

There are three basic facts about regarding sunlight and skin cancer that you need to know:

1) Long-term, excessive exposure to sunlight can increase the risk of non-melanoma skin cancer, although regular, moderate sun exposure is actually less dangerous than intermittent sun exposure.

2) Sunburns can also increase the risk of melanoma, but there is little to no evidence that sun exposure without sunburn increases melanoma risk.

3) There is a good deal of evidence that sun exposure without sunburns significantly *decreases* the risk of melanoma.

Let's start by putting things in perspective a bit. Melanoma is typically a type of skin cancer which is frequently fatal if left untreated. But we need to put this into the proper perspective. Non-melanoma skin cancer has a very low death rate; fewer than half of one percent of those who develop non-melanoma skin cancer die, which works out to about 1,200 people each year in the U.S.[1]

1,200 people is only two-tenths of one percent of all annual U.S. cancer deaths. It amounts to a twentieth of a percent of yearly U.S. deaths from all causes. You are more than four times more likely to die of food poisoning. You are more than 653 times more likely to be accidentally killed by your doctor as a result of medical errors.[2]

It might be advisable to keep that in mind the next time you are told that "sunlight causes cancer."

What Causes Melanoma?

Melanoma, on the other hand, is far more dangerous because it has the potential to metastasize very quickly. This means that the cancer does not stay in the skin, but spreads through the blood and lymph system to bones and organs, such as the brain, lungs, and liver.

Melanoma risk increases in association with sunburns, rising along with their frequency and severity. The effect is particularly pronounced for childhood sunburns. However, there is little to no evidence that long-term sun exposure without sunburn will lead to melanoma. In fact, study after study has shown that precisely the opposite is true.

When melanomas do occur, they usually do so on parts of the body that receive little or no sun exposure. In men, melanoma most often appears on the upper back, and in women it is usually seen on the legs. If melanoma were primarily caused by sunlight, one would expect it to appear more often on the face and hands; that is where non-melanoma skin cancer tends to develop. Melanoma can also develop in locations other than the skin, including sites such as the rectum, vulva, vagina, mouth, respiratory tract, gastro-intestinal tract, and bladder, most of which either receive little sunlight or cannot be exposed to sunlight at all.

Of particular interest is that melanoma is seen more often in those who do not receive regular sunlight, than those who do. A landmark study by Doctors Cedric and Frank Garland, for example, demonstrated that Navy personnel who worked above decks on aircraft carriers actually developed melanomas less often than those who worked below decks.[3] Sailors who worked both indoors and outdoors had the lowest incidence of the disease, bearing out the notion that while sunburn can be a causative factor, regular sunlight prevents it.

A number of more recent studies have revealed much the same result; in 2004 and 2005, for example, a pair of large European studies demonstrated that sunlight and UV radiation, without sunburn, were not causative factors in melanoma, and in fact offered some degree of protection against it.[4,5]

What's more, it is well known among scientists, although often not widely mentioned, that melanoma actually increases among those who regularly use sunscreen. In 1992, Frank and Cedric Garland noted that, "Worldwide, the countries where chemical sunscreens have been recommended and adopted have experienced the greatest rise in malignant melanoma."[6]

Sunlight and Other Forms of Cancer

The effects of sunlight on melanoma are not particularly surprising to anyone familiar with the research. Sunlight has, in fact, been shown to protect against as many as sixteen different types of cancer, including breast, colon, endometrial, esophageal, ovarian, bladder, gallbladder, gastric, pancreatic, prostate, rectal, and renal cancers, as well as non-Hodgkin's lymphoma.[7]

One of the earliest statistical studies of cancer, which looked at large cities throughout the world, showed a striking correlation between deaths from cancer of all types and distance from the equator, where sunshine is strongest, as outlined in the chart below.

Mortality from Cancer (per 100,000 People) in Large Cities, by Latitude[8]

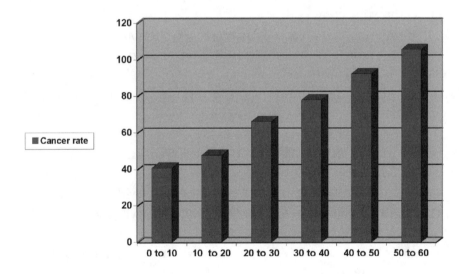

Degrees Latitude

Sunlight's anti-cancer effects come primarily from the fact that it stimulates your body to produce vitamin D. Many researchers are

153

currently evaluating vitamin D and its analogs in the treatment of a number of different cancers. The connection in the research studies is borne out time and time again.

What Is Vitamin D?

Although vitamin D is called a vitamin, it is more accurately classified as a hormone. Vitamins are substances that cannot be produced by your body, but must instead be ingested in the diet. Although you can take vitamin D orally in pills or cod liver oil, the primary form in which you receive it is through sun exposure on your skin. However hormones can be produced independently by your body.

Like all hormones, vitamin D is part of a family of chemicals called steroids (a family is a group of chemicals with similar molecular structures). Other steroids include cortisone and cholesterol. In fact, vitamin D is very closely related to cholesterol, and both are created by the transformation of the chemical squalene, which is naturally present in your body.

Hormones act as chemical messengers, controlling such processes as growth, sexual maturation, reproduction, and blood glucose levels. They work by actually turning segments of your DNA on and off and signaling your cells to produce a variety of proteins and enzymes.

Ultraviolet (UV) light stimulates a chemical process in your skin that produces vitamin D. Wearing sunscreen actually blocks your body's production of vitamin D. A sunscreen of only SPF 8 will reduce your vitamin D production by 97.5 percent, and an SPF 15 sunscreen will reduce it by 99.9 percent.[9] Even without sunscreen, UV light is not always strong enough to stimulate vitamin D production. Latitude and time of year, as well as time of day, can have an enormous effect on this. For example, for four to five months in the winter, it is nearly impossible to produce any significant vitamin D from sunlight in the Boston area.[10]

The MOST Potent Hormone In Your Body

In the kidneys, vitamin D helps maintain your blood calcium levels. For many years, it was believed that this function, along with phosphate metabolism, was the primary purpose of vitamin D and that your kidneys were the only organ that contained receptors that could convert vitamin D to an active form. However, more recently, it has been shown that vitamin D receptors exist in tissues throughout your body and they have nothing to do with calcium or phosphate regulation. In those tissues, vitamin D signals your genes to produce hundreds of crucial enzymes and proteins, affecting your body's organs, systems, and health in hundreds of different ways.

This is relatively new information and it is likely that physicians who graduated from medical school later than 2005 would not be aware of it.

This means that vitamin D has a function in nearly every part of your body. Since the discovery that vitamin D receptors are present in so many bodily tissues, the evidence has been pouring in regarding the many, many uses and benefits of vitamin D. In fact, vitamin D is by far the most potent steroid hormone in the human body. It is active in quantities as small as $1/1,000,000,000,000$ of a gram.

Vitamin D And Cancer

There are thousands of studies supporting the role of vitamin D in cancer; the evidence is absolutely overwhelming. So much so that it should be considered malpractice that vitamin D levels are not measured on every single cancer patient. This is something that we do for all our patients at the Optimal Wellness Center, but if you or someone you know struggles with cancer, it is vital that you share this information with them as it could literally be the difference between life and death.

Both cancer incidence and cancer mortality rates are affected by your vitamin D level. A recent review of no fewer than 63 studies on the subject found that the "evidence suggests that efforts to improve vitamin D status . . . could reduce cancer incidence and mortality at low cost, with few or no adverse effects."[11]

The list of cancer types affected by sunlight and vitamin D is nearly endless. A recent report, based on findings from 1966–2004, indicates that vitamin D can reduce the risk of breast cancer by as much as 50 percent.[12]

Studies have also shown that men with higher levels of vitamin D in their blood were half as likely to develop aggressive forms of prostate cancer.[13] An eight-year study of more than 25,000 people conducted in the 1980's found that people who had normal vitamin D levels reduced their risk of colon cancer by *80 percent*.[14] Vitamin D has been shown to have preventive or protective effects against leukemia, lung cancer, kidney cancer, thyroid cancer, ovarian cancer, pancreatic cancer, non-Hodgkin's lymphoma, and many other forms of cancer as well.[15]

Vitamin D And Your Health

Cancer is only one of a laundry list of ailments that vitamin D reduces the effects of, protects against, or outright prevents. It helps maintain your health your whole life long; studies have even shown that elderly men and women who are deficient in vitamin D are significantly more likely to be admitted to a nursing home than those with high levels of the vitamin.[16]

Some of vitamin D's functions are fairly well-known to the general public; others have only been hinted at in a few promising studies. But given how vital vitamin D is to every part of your body, even the benefits presented in this chapter are likely only a fraction of the ways in which vitamin D keeps you healthy and fit.

- Vitamin D has been shown to have a positive, protective, or healing action on ailments as diverse as: Autoimmune disorders (including rheumatoid arthritis, inflammatory bowel disease, multiple sclerosis, and type I diabetes)[17]
- Cardiovascular disease[18]
- Blood pressure[19]
- High cholesterol levels[20]
- Neurological disorders (including Parkinson's disease, Alzheimer's disease, and even schizophrenia)[21]

156

- Disorders of the reproductive system (including Polycystic Ovary Syndrome, PMS, and infertility)[22]
- Kidney failure[23]
- Muscle Weakness[24]
- Skin diseases (such as eczema and psoriasis)[25]
- And even tooth decay![26]

Vitamin D and Bone Health

Vitamin D's best-known property is very likely the role it plays in maintaining healthy bones. Most everyone is aware that vitamin D plays an important role in keeping bones strong.

Vitamin D sends messages to your intestines to increase the absorption of calcium (as well as phosphorus). Vitamin D not only helps to form and maintain bones by promoting calcium absorption, but also works in concert with a number of other vitamins, minerals, and hormones to promote bone mineralization. Without vitamin D, bones can become thin, brittle, or misshapen. Vitamin D sufficiency prevents rickets in children and osteomalacia in adults, two forms of skeletal diseases that weaken bones. Vitamin D can also help prevent the onset of osteoporosis and help to alleviate it if it has already occurred.[27]

Vitamin D and Infectious Disease

The relationship between sunlight and relief from infectious diseases has been known for quite some time. Two Nobel prizes were awarded in the early twentieth century to physicians who used sunlight as a treatment for tuberculosis, and sunlight was used to successfully cure illnesses long before the advent of antibiotics.[28]

A bounty of recent evidence has strongly suggested that vitamin D is the primary causative factor in such cures. Vitamin D is a potent antibiotic. It works primarily by increasing your body's production of proteins called antimicrobial peptides. Antimicrobial peptides destroy the cell walls of bacteria, fungi, and viruses.

In April 2005, an influenza epidemic started sweeping through the maximum-security hospital for the criminally insane where Dr. John Cannell worked. But as the epidemic progressed, he noticed something unusual: although wards all around his became infected, no patients on his ward became ill, despite intermingling of both patients and nurses. The only difference was that all of the patients on Dr. Cannell's ward had been taking 2,000 units of vitamin D every day.[29]

It is interesting to note that the high doses of vitamin D used on Dr. Cannell's patients have been shown to have effects which could be as potent as the "miracle" antibiotics on which modern medicine largely depends. Doses up to 600,000 units are routinely used in Europe in a treatment called "Stoss" therapy, which is used to treat acute infection or vitamin D deficiency. However, it should be noted that it would be unwise to use such high oral doses as a regular program due to the risk of oral vitamin D overdose.

After observing the effects of the vitamin on his patients, Dr. Cannell posited that the antimicrobial properties of vitamin D could explain why the flu predictably occurs in the months following the winter solstice in temperate regions, and why influenza is more common in the tropics during the rainy season; there is less sunlight exposure during those times. It could also explain why children exposed to sunlight are less likely to get colds, and why the elderly who live in countries with high vitamin D consumption, like Norway, are less likely to die in the winter than people in countries at similar latitudes where vitamin D consumption is not as high.[30]

These same observations on the seasonality of influenza led the famed epidemiologist Dr. R. Edward Hope-Simpson to a startling conclusion. After conducting study after study, he postulated that rather than being primarily spread person-to-person, vitamin D deficiency occurring in the less sunny months was rendering people vulnerable to a latent virus. In fact, he concluded that vitamin D deficiency was the major factor behind influenza epidemics![31]

This is a stunning idea. If the spread of influenza, or other epidemic diseases, is actually largely a matter of vitamin D deficiency, then it is possible that epidemics that kill millions could be avoided simply by means of sunlight and sensible supplementation.

158

Can Sunshine Help You Normalize Your Weight?

Getting your weight under control is one of the most important things you can do for your long-term physical health. The current obesity epidemic has come about as a result of poor dietary and lifestyle choices. Simply eating less processed foods and becoming more active will do wonders for your body. But recent evidence also points to another, less obvious, means of normalizing your weight—vitamin D.

Low vitamin D is a consistent predictor of obesity, and some studies have flat-out shown that the more vitamin D in your diet, the less you are likely to weigh.[32] The likely reason is that vitamin D lowers leptin secretion. Leptin is a hormone produced by fat cells, and it is involved in weight regulation. Vitamin D and calcium have also been shown to work in concert to control fat metabolism.[33]

Vitamin D is deposited in your body fat, meaning that in over-weight people, it becomes less available to the rest of your body. This can become a vicious cycle; obesity hastens vitamin D deficiency, which in turn increases obesity.

If you are one of the two-thirds of people in developed countries who are overweight or obese then maintaining a normal body weight is clearly one of your health goals and spending adequate time outside should be added to your list of healthy behaviors, alongside regular exercise and a healthy diet.

What Is The BEST Way To Supplement With Vitamin D?

Many of you, reading this chapter, may be wondering why sunlight is necessary, if the truly important factor is vitamin D. Why not just pop a multivitamin or vitamin D capsule and not worry about how much time you spend in the sun?

First, there are benefits to sunlight in addition to vitamin D, such as the neurological and psychological benefits of full-spectrum sunlight, which will be detailed later on in the chapter. But also, most experts agree that sunlight is far and away the best way to get vitamin D. When sunlight strikes your skin, you generate enough vitamin D for effective use with virtually no risk of overdosing. Your body will stop producing vitamin D before you produce potentially toxic levels. In effect, this makes it difficult to overdose on vitamin D obtained from sunlight.

The same cannot be said for any other kind of vitamin D supplementation. About the only way you can overdose on vitamin D with sun exposure is if you had been consuming oral vitamin D. I did this on one of my winter trips to Maui. I had taken cod liver oil for November and December in Chicago, and when I returned in March to check my vitamin D levels, the level was one of the highest we ever measured. Vitamin D excess can cause the same symptoms as a vitamin D deficiency.

Fortunately, excessive vitamin D levels produced from sun exposure decrease far more rapidly than excessive vitamin D levels from oral sources. My level normalized within a few weeks. Had I overdosed on vitamin D with no sun exposure, with those levels it could have easily been a year before my levels normalized, and nothing short of time or hemodialysis (a machine that removes waste products from the blood) would lower it any sooner.

However, most people will not have regular access to sun exposure on their skin in the winter, so supplementation of some kind is necessary. As has already been mentioned, in many latitudes distant from the equator, it is virtually impossible to generate enough vitamin D from sunlight during the winter months. But even then, it is important to realize that not all vitamin D is the same.

Different Types of Oral Vitamin D

Supplemental vitamin D comes in two forms: ergocalciferol (vitamin D2) and cholecalciferol (vitamin D3). These have generally been regarded as equivalent and interchangeable, but that idea is based on studies more than seventy years old. Vitamin D3 is the form found in natural food sources; vitamin D2 is an artificial form originally created by exposing certain foods, such as milk, to ultraviolet light.

Recent studies have shown that vitamin D3 is much more potent; vitamin D2 has a shorter shelf life, and its metabolites bind with protein poorly, making it less effective. Vitamin D3 is converted into an active form 500 percent faster than vitamin D2. And, while there have been no clinical trials to date demonstrating conclusively that D2 helps to prevent bone fractures, every clinical trial of D3 has shown it does.[34]

However, the form of vitamin D used in most multi-vitamins and supplements in North America is vitamin D2. Vitamin D2 is also used in fortified milk. The reason is unsurprising; since vitamin D2 is generated by an unnatural process, it can be patented and licensed for use in products. Once again, greed has resulted in a less healthy version of a substance becoming the more commonly used one.

The best way to supplement the vitamin D you obtain from sunlight is with natural food sources, such as cod liver oil. D3-containing cod liver oil has been shown to be four times as effective as Viosterol, a medicinal preparation of vitamin D2.[35] Vitamin D also has therapeutic levels of vitamin A which help minimize any potential vitamin D toxicity.

TAKE CONTROL

Recovery From a Potentially Fatal Autoimmune Problem

I was so sick that I could barely pick up my 15 lb baby boy or a gallon of milk. I couldn't even climb stairs due to weak legs. I had a red itchy rash all over my face, neck and chest, and my right knee resembled having a second-degree burn. This caused restless sleep and I was constantly tired. Testing showed that I had dermatomyositis, an autoimmune disease that causes muscle myopathy. My doctor's prognosis was grim, and his course of treatment was high doses of Prednisone and Fosamax. I scheduled a consultation with Dr. Mercola. His course of treatment was to eliminate grains, sugar and dairy from my diet, and add lots of raw foods, cod liver oil and healthy sources of protein. I used EFT to help with the diet. Real improvement showed within three months. Soon, I was the model of good health! I no longer take any medications, my strength and energy have returned, and the rash is almost gone.

—*Suzanne Delich, Dyer, Indiana* ❧

However, I must emphasize that even this should only be done under supervision by a health care professional who can monitor your vitamin D levels. Remember that vitamin D in excessive doses can be toxic and cause complications similar to vitamin D deficiency. Excessive doses of vitamin D can cause calcium to deposit in your soft tissues and kidney. I do not advise oral supplements of any kind, not even cod liver oil, unless you can have your blood levels regularly monitored. However, most can tolerate small doses of cod liver oil during the winter months if they are not going to have any sun exposure   The other option to consider in the winter months is regular exposure to safe forms of tanning booths, which I discuss in more detail in a moment.

Vitamin D, Infants, and Pregnancy

Vitamin D is the only "vitamin" recommended as a supplement for newborn infants whose skin is not regularly exposed to the sun. This is because breast milk, in all other respects the perfect food for infants, contains very little vitamin D. However, it would be incorrect to take this to mean that breast milk is somehow "deficient" because of this lack. Human infants are designed to get their vitamin D from sunlight and only require supplementation if they live at higher latitudes or climates which don't get much sun, or are kept indoors for much of the time.

Less than optimal bone development, including the possibility of rickets and other problems, can occur without adequate vitamin D. Parents are typically concerned about calcium for proper bone growth and health, but in most cases, proper sun exposure and vitamin D is far more important. Young children who receive the least supplemental vitamin D are also at a five-fold higher risk for developing type 1 diabetes later in life,[36] and male children who receive little vitamin D also suffer a similarly higher risk of developing schizophrenia later on.[37]

My recommendation for the best form of supplementation for infants who are not regularly exposed to sunshine is once again cod liver oil. Breast-fed infants really seem to benefit from cod liver oil. Not much is needed—typically about 1 cc or ml for every ten pounds of body weight. If the baby refuses to swallow it, the cod liver oil can even be rubbed on the skin and the absorption will be nearly as good.

Vitamin D levels are also important for the developing fetus during pregnancy. Several studies have found that the birth size and height of an infant are related to the amount of sunlight the mother receives during pregnancy.[38]

There is also mounting evidence that suggests that vitamin D deficiency during pregnancy can alter the development of a child's brain in the womb; for example, people who develop schizophrenia in Europe and North America have been shown to be more likely to have been born in the spring (i.e., a winter pregnancy), and winter pregnancies have also been shown to be 700 percent more likely to result in learning disabilities in children.[39] Other research has determined that severe maternal vitamin D deficiency permanently damages the brains of baby rats, and even transient vitamin D deficiency can lead to neurological birth defects.[40]

Other Psychological and Neurological Benefits of Sunlight

Vitamin D is not the only benefit derived from sunlight. Throughout most of human history we have lived according to the constant, once-daily cycle of light and darkness, day and night. Your body and brain, therefore, adapted to this rhythm, which is called the circadian rhythm. You are meant to wake as the daylight brightens and fall asleep during the dark of night.

As I will cover more thoroughly in Chapter Twelve on sleep, this rhythm has been disrupted for many people in the modern era, and this can be dangerous for your health. Many studies have shown that night-shift workers are more prone to cancer, and that those who work on rotating shifts are in even more danger still, even if they have sufficient vitamin D levels.[41] The electric light bulb is rightly hailed as one of the most transformative inventions of all time, but it also can, and has, indirectly cost many people their health. When you do not sleep and wake in the correct cycle, or are only exposed to poor substitutes for the full-spectrum rays of the sun during daylight hours, your body's delicate balance of hormones and neurotransmitters becomes disrupted.

When you are asleep, and your eyes detect an increased level of light (even when they are closed), a signal is sent to your brain's pineal gland. The pineal gland then triggers the production of the hormone serotonin, which causes you to slowly awaken. This natural method of waking leaves you feeling refreshed and energized.

At the other end of the circadian scale, in response to darkness, your pineal gland triggers the production of the hormone melatonin. So, if you are exposed to light during your normal sleep hours, your production of melatonin can be radically reduced, and if this occurs on a regular basis, you will clearly increase your risk of cancer as melatonin is a very potent cancer-regulating hormone.

One common result of insufficient daylight is a form of depression that occurs when the days shorten in the winter called seasonal affective disorder or SAD. People with seasonal affective disorder shift their melatonin levels with the seasons, paralleling the hibernation patterns of mammals. In patients with SAD, the duration of melatonin secretion becomes longer in winter and shorter in summer, just as it occurs in other mammals. But when the sleep/wake schedule does not also change to match this, the neurological changes can trigger depression.

For many people, it is impractical to alter their schedule completely as the seasons change. Some methods have been found, however, to artificially replicate the experience of waking with the sun and sleeping during the darkness.

Bright light treatments (exposure to special light boxes that replicate sunlight) are the recommended treatment for SAD. They are especially effective when administered first thing in the morning. Special alarm clocks that simulate the effects of dawn breaking have also been shown to help alleviate the symptoms of SAD.

Tanning Beds

Tanning beds use UV rays which will increase your vitamin D levels. But they do not provide the aforementioned neurological and psychological benefits of the sun's full-spectrum light. I do not recommend conventional tanning beds, because the humming noise that you hear when you lie on a tanning bed is the magnetic ballast which emits huge amounts of electromagnetic frequency (EMF) radiation. EMF can potentially cause brain tumors, leukemia, birth defects, miscarriages, chronic fatigue, headaches, cataracts, heart problems, stress, nausea, chest pain, forgetfulness, and cancer. In a draft report, the EPA recommended that EMF be classified as a potential human carcinogen although heavy lobbying by businesses prevented that classification from becoming official.[42]

However, it is possible to construct a "safe" tanning bed, by removing the magnetic ballast and replacing it with a quiet and much more efficient electronic ballast. I produced a video on this on the site along with more detailed information with a list of some tanning facilities across the country that use this type of equipment.

For more information, go to http://www.mercola.com/2006/nov/11/can-a-tanning-bed-be-healthy.htm

The Myth of Sunblock

Although you should take care not to get burned, most sunscreens should be avoided and are one of the last things you should put on your body; what's more, it's not even a good way to limit sun exposure if you need to do so. Ideally it is best to use strategically placed clothing to limit sun exposure.

Most sunscreens contain toxic chemicals that can cause health problems and increase your risk of disease. The main chemical used in sun lotions to filter out UVB light, octyl methoxycinnamate (OMC), was found to kill mouse cells even at low doses.[43] OMC, ironically enough, was shown to be particularly toxic when exposed to sunshine. OMC is present in 90 percent of sunscreen brands. A common UVA filter, butyl methoxydibenzoylmethane, has also been shown to have toxic properties.[44]

Even if sunscreen didn't contribute to disease, studies have shown that sunscreen does not protect against melanoma.[45] However, there are some safe sunscreens on the market using the ingredient titanium dioxide.

Safe Sun Exposure

None of this means you should simply go out and get as much sun as you want, as excessive sun exposure can clearly be problematic. You must exercise caution and be careful not to burn. At the beginning of the season, go out gradually and limit your exposure to perhaps as little as

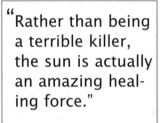

"Rather than being a terrible killer, the sun is actually an amazing healing force."

10 minutes a day. Progressively increase your time in the sun so that in a few weeks, you will be able to have normal sun exposure with little risk of skin cancer.

You may also need to vary the amount of time you spend in the sun based on your skin type. The paler your skin, the more quickly you will burn. If you have very pale skin, you will need to increase your tolerance to the sun very slowly.

You can further avoid the damage from the sun by staying out of the sun during the most potentially damaging times, from 10 AM to 2 PM, especially if you are just starting a new summer or vacation season. You can stay in the shade during this time or wear lightweight long-sleeved shirts, long pants, and a wide-brimmed hat.

Be very careful to avoid sunburn. That is the key.

In Conclusion

You are likely to encounter skepticism from others when you start to put the principles found in this chapter into practice. The myth of the dangerous sun is deeply ingrained in the current culture; it has had decades of reinforcement from the media and powerful corporate interests. Be assured that for the immediate future if you attempt to apply the information in this chapter you will most likely be told that you are putting your health, or your children's health, at risk; that you will damage your body irreparably; even that you will die an early death.

We urge you to treat this as what it is—alarmism. Your body evolved for hundreds of generations under the sun's rays. For most of history, your ancestors have been outdoors far more often than they were indoors. How is it possible that your body could have ended up configured in such a way that the sun was a deadly force to us? It would be like being allergic to air. How could we have survived, as a species, if we were that vulnerable to something humans have been exposed to constantly for nearly their entire existence? This is a perversion of rational logic and simply makes no sense. And it makes no sense because it quite simply isn't true.

Rather than being a terrible killer, the sun is actually an amazing healing force. Sunlight is the ultimate source of the energy in the food chain. Indeed, without the energy of the sun, all life would cease to exist. After reading this chapter, my hope is that you will no longer fear the sun, but look to it as an essential supplier of wonderful vitamin D.

CHAPTER:

Your Emotional Health
The Foundation of Your Physical Health

Having positive *emotional* and *mental well being* is **vital** for having optimal *physical* health. This is because, far from being two separate entities, your mind and your body are constantly interacting and, in fact, are so intertwined that they directly impact one another.

Some of the connections between your mind and your body are obvious. For example, anxiety may lead to the physical experience of nausea, chest pain, or diarrhea. Depression can lead to fatigue and low appetite. Other connections, such as those between stress, negative emotions, and disease, are not quite so forthright, but still they're there.

Negative Emotions Are a Major Cause of Illness

In the three decades that I have practiced medicine, it has been my consistent experience that most illness has an emotional component that needs to be addressed for complete healing to occur. My colleague Carol Tuttle, who is an energy therapist, also has extensive practice in helping people improve their health and well being by clearing emotional issues. We combined our experience and knowledge in mind-body medicine to write this chapter.

An astounding number of research studies have found concrete links between negative emotions and disease. For instance:

- People with symptoms of depression have a lower immune response[1] (which indicates they're less able to fight off disease)

- Women who are hostile during arguments with their spouse have a greater risk of heart disease, as do men who behave in a dominating or controlling manner[2]

- Engaging in arguments makes it take longer for physical wounds to heal[3]

- Pessimists tend to have worse health over the long-term than their optimistic peers[4]

Even the highly conservative U.S. Centers of Disease Control and Prevention (CDC) states that **up to 90% of doctor visits** in the United States are triggered by a stress-related illness.

The good news, however, is that the opposite also holds true. Just as negative emotions can hinder your health, positive emotions can support it and help it flourish. Consider these findings:

- Positive emotions may help keep your blood pressure at a healthy level[5]

- Meditation is known to produce beneficial changes in the brain and immune system[6]

- Being optimistic may increase physical health and mental functioning

- Laughing may boost the immune system and reduce inflammation

Your Thoughts and Feelings Are Energy Vibrations

To delve into the mind-body connection a bit deeper, it helps to think of your thoughts and feelings as energy. After all, everything, at its finest level of creation is energy. You are exchanging energy and silently communicating energetically with every person you meet or come into contact with. Believe it or not, energy impressions are typically your first impressions—the ones that influence what you think or feel about others.

Your thoughts and feelings create a frequency that flows through your own physical body as well. Everything you see, hear, feel, taste, and smell is permanently recorded in your brain and transmitted along your nervous system through complex electrochemical messages in your energy system. If you touch a hot stove, you feel pain due to the nerve endings in your hand sending instantaneous electrochemical messages through your nerves to your brain. (This electrical system is essential to your physical health and without it you would die.)

Similarly, when you encounter a traumatic emotional experience, it is also recorded in your body. However, these recordings have far more potential to cause you physical damage than touching a hot stove has. A burn on your finger is only temporary and then it heals, but an emotional trauma, stored in your body, can cause a chronic disruption of your body's energy system. This disruption often leads to disease or "dis-ease."

It is in this way that positive thoughts and feelings produce biochemical changes in the body that enhance your health. Negative thoughts and feelings can produce biochemical changes that damage your health, such as an impaired immune system or chronic disease.

Much has been written about the correlation between physical health and emotional and mental influences. Louise Hay has been a pioneer in mind-body medicine and has written extensively on the emotional origin of physical diseases in her book: *Heal Your Body*. It is a valuable and quick reference guide that can assist you in discovering your negative patterns. In her book, Hay teaches:

> The mental thought patterns that cause the most disease in the body are: criticism, anger, resentment and guilt. For instance, criticism indulged in long enough will often lead to diseases such as arthritis. Anger turns into things that boil and burn and infect the body.
>
> Resentment long held festers and eats away all the self and ultimately can lead to tumors and cancer. Guilt always

seeks punishment and leads to pain. It is so much easier to release these negative emotional and mental patterns with the clearing technologies and healing arts we have available to us today, when we are healthy, than to wait until we are in a physical crisis and our body has deteriorated considerably.[7]

Many people have, in fact, healed their health challenges simply by clearing up their negative energies and thinking patterns, and you can too.

Carol Tuttle used Louise Hay's book *Heal Your Body* to identify the emotional contributors to her health problem. Carol recalls:

In my early forties, I discovered a substantial lump in my breast. I told my husband and asked him not to make a big deal about it. I went to the doctor and she told me I should get a mammogram within the week. I made the decision at this point that I was not going to tell anyone because I did not want attention put on the worst-case scenario. I was also aware a part of me thought it would be nice to get a lot of attention and concern from others. So, I told no one, and proceeded instead to understand my emotional/mental relationship to this disharmony.

I learned by reading *Heal Your Body*, that breast lumps were generated from fear of letting go of your children, over mothering patterns, and over bearing attitudes as a parent. I certainly did not like to think of myself this way. Rather than resist it, I accepted the possibility that this was my stuff and asked God to let me know how to change this.

I noticed that my oldest daughter was beginning to date and maybe I was a little too emotionally involved. Therapists can be overbearing with their children, because they think they are helping them with so many answers. I was willing to change all that. I thanked my body for the message and started a new thought pattern that sounded like this:

I am perfect just as God created me. I believe I am important and I make a difference. I know when to speak and when to keep quiet. I am allowing my children to be who they are. We are all safe and free.

Continued on next page

Continued from page 159

The first mammogram identified the lump as either a tumor or a cyst. Another test identified it as a benign cyst. My doctor encouraged me to have it surgically removed. My appointment with a surgeon was six weeks after the mammogram. During that time, I did visualizations, imagining white laser light clearing out the cyst. I continued repeating my new beliefs and noticed when I was overbearing with my children and stopped myself. When I went for my appointment with the surgeon, the cyst was gone.

Why We Hold on to Disease and Disharmony

Sometimes, people will unconsciously manifest a disease condition in order to get their needs met. When we become aware of the value these patterns provide us, we are then free to let them go and meet our needs in healthy ways.

TAKE CONTROL

Kathy had been diagnosed with chronic fatigue. In just a few sessions, she discovered she had a belief that she was not lovable unless she was doing something to make her feel worthwhile. She was a classic overachiever and did not know how to give herself a break. There was a Little Kathy inside her that believed she did not measure up and could never do anything well enough.

She had to keep trying with no rest. Her chronic fatigue condition was what she manifested to give herself permission to let go and take a break. She needed the condition because she was unable to give herself this permission without it.

In her sessions, she easily cleared the old emotions and beliefs, formed new ones, and changed her behavior patterns—taking time to sit and meditate each day.

She verbally acknowledged her self-worth, vitality, and energy. She now holds the belief, "I am worthwhile and loved, I choose to do what is inspired action in my life. All that I do is good enough and I am experiencing other people knowing that about me." ❧

Therefore, if you have a disease condition, it is important to avoid making your disease part of your identity. It is common for people who have been diagnosed with a condition to say:

"I am a diabetic."

"I have attention deficit."

"I have chronic fatigue."

"I am overweight."

"I am depressed."

"I am a survivor of sexual abuse."

"I am manic depressive," and many other physical, mental and emotional ailments. But by saying "I am" they are directing their body and all its cells to confirm that "this is my identity, so act accordingly."

TAKE CONTROL

Andrea had been experiencing many years of bad health. Nothing very dramatic, she was just always getting sick. In her sessions she discovered that when she was a little girl she received a little more attention when she was ill. We worked with a 5-year old part of her that did not want to give up being sick; in fact it was the 5-year old's job to attract illnesses just so Andrea would receive love and support. In her adult life there was always a doctor or nurse who would listen to her and want to help her feel better.

Andrea believed that without the illnesses she might not get any love and attention. Like many others, I (Carol Tuttle) have worked with. Her deepest fear was that she might discover that she was really inferior and inadequate and no one would want to love her. With this possibility in her deeper mind, she was afraid to let go of the substitute she had created. I said to her, "So you think if we go deep within you, I am going to discover the real truth about you which would sound something like this: 'I am sorry, Andrea, but it seems you really are inadequate and unlovable. You did come into this life less than everyone else; there is nothing I can do for you. Good luck as you continue to survive as a lesser human being with a flawed spirit!'"

When they hear their deepest fears expressed, people usually realize how ridiculous their fears are and have a good laugh. They begin to trust that as we start clearing away the layers of lies, they will find a love for themselves that will bring them to their knees in gratitude. Many clients begin to feel this self-love in their first session. ❧

"I am" statements are the most powerful expression of telling your body what you believe your identity is. Remember, you control your mind; your mind, to a large extent, controls your body.

A healthy expression, one that supports you in overcoming disharmonies, is:

> My body has experienced the condition of _____ in the past, and now I choose to get the message it has for me, clear the disharmonies, claim my real self, and move on.

This statement, rather than identifying yourself with the disease, accurately describes the situation without making it your current identity, puts it in the past, takes responsibility for clearing the disharmonies causing the imbalance, and exercises faith to heal.

The Secret and the Law of Attraction

At the beginning of 2007, a film called *The Secret* began to gather much attention (it was featured on Oprah and was number one on many of the bestseller lists). *The Secret* expands on an important principle of energy psychology, which is the **Law of Attraction**. In simple terms, the Law of Attraction means that whatever you put your focus and attention on, you tend to manifest in your life.

How Does The *Law of Attraction* Work?

Remember, every time you verbalize, in private or in public, that you don't deserve this or that, or you complain about life circumstances that you don't want, or that you feel sick, or that you can never get well, your biology will hear it and act accordingly. What do you want to tell yourself?

Every person has an electromagnetic field with a vibration that sends a signal out into the world. By thinking thoughts that make you feel good, you increase your vibration. You are constantly sending messages out to the world with what you think, feel, and say. There is one guarantee with the Law of Attraction, and that is that everything you put out returns to you—multiplied. If you think, feel, and talk a lot about being sick and tired, you will multiply the energy and create more experiences of feeling sick and tired.

Creating a strong intention in which you can hold a belief is the most powerful way to use your thoughts. Intentions are decisions, goals, ideas, wants, desires, and choices that are stated in the affirmative. Whatever you put your faith in will be your life experience. When you match your intentions with a positive feeling of hope, you send a signal out to the world that is honored, and you receive what you have intended.

As you make decisions each day about what you want to experience, you set into motion the creation of that experience. You are the one who literally molds your future experience. As you set thoughts of what you want into motion, in combination with the excited emotion, you will be in a perfect position to receive that which you desire. The more specific you are about what you want, the more specifically you will receive that which you want. The more vague you are in stating what you want, the more vaguely you will receive that which you want.

What keeps you from believing with absolute certainty that you have the ability to manifest whatever you want in life? Often it is your pessimism that you will not get what you want, and you will be disappointed. You may believe that God is in charge and it is up to Him if you are to have something. What if God gives you full reign to create whatever you choose for your experience and all you have to do is make a choice and think, say, and behave as if that choice were already a part of your reality?

Another common stumbling block that prevents people from using the Law of Attraction is that people expect the worst. If you are one of these people, you must ask yourself, *"Why do you choose that thought?"* Most explain, *"Because then I am prepared when bad things happen, or I can prevent the worst from happening."* But if you think about worst case scenarios, you are setting yourself up for the worst to happen. The greatest power you have in avoiding the worst is to intend for the best to happen. Ask yourself, *"If everything were going your way in this situation, what would be the ideal experience for you?"* Most people cannot imagine the ideal because they have been programmed to believe that it cannot happen for them.

When things go wrong in your life, it is helpful to take full responsibility and ask the following questions:

- Why am I creating this?
- Am I attracting this into my life?
- What can I learn from it?

These questions can be followed by:

- What do I really want?
- If the ideal thing happened in this situation, what would that look like? For me?

Take the power of your mind, the power of your thoughts, and start creating the life you really want. Catch yourself thinking the worst and ask yourself in that moment, *"If I could have anything I want in this situation, what would that look like?"*

If you really believe you deserve something and believe it can happen, it can. If you doubt it, question it, or keep your attention on what has still not happened for you, you will most likely not receive it.

Most people wish that at least one area of their lives was better than how it currently is. They wish they had better health, or more money, or more harmonious relationships, or a more fulfilling job. Unfortunately, people tend to focus on *what they don't want* which only brings them **more** of what they don't want.

They might say:

"I've always been overweight and I guess I always will be. Nothing I've tried has worked long term."

"I have so much debt; I'll always be broke!"

But, if they want to be in a relationship or be prosperous, they have to say things like:

"I am a slim 150 pounds and I love my new healthy lifestyle."

"I am making $75,000 a year and all my debts are paid off."

Even if the above statements aren't true yet, they are messages you are sending to your own brain and to the universe that will help you obtain what you want.

Resources to Help You Achieve Optimum Emotional and Mental Health

While very few would dispute the statement that a healthy mind and healthy emotions contribute to a healthy body, very few health professionals have proper training on how to address their patients' emotional issues. Physicians, for example, are not trained in medical school to explore the emotional issues contributing to patients' physical illness.

If you have an obvious emotional problem such as chronic anxiety or depression, the overwhelming majority of physicians will prescribe psychotropic drugs like antidepressants and anti-anxiety agents, which come with potentially life-threatening side effects (such as suicide). These drugs in no way, shape, or form treat the underlying cause of disease.

If you don't want to take a drug, then the other main choice in the United States is to get some therapy to talk about your issues, your childhood, and everything else that is seemingly related. While this may be beneficial for some, this approach typically fails to heal the underlying disruption in your body's energy system.

Thankfully, we have a tool that does. It is a revolutionary breakthrough in mind-body medicine called **Energy Psychology**.

Energy psychology is a family of mind/body techniques that have been proven to help with a wide range of psychological conditions.

The field of Energy Psychology rests on the principle that disruptions in your body's energy system can lead to negative emotions and physical health problems. Therefore, it uses techniques that work with *energy* pathways (acupuncture points), energy centers (chakras) and the systems of energy that envelop the body to help you clear the negative energy that creates imbalances in your physical system. Working on all three levels (mind, body, and energetic) means that energy psychology can be more effective than conventional talk therapy. After years and years of talk therapy I've seen patients who have resolved long standing problems in one session of energy psychology.

One huge advantage of learning one of these techniques is that you can do them yourself any time you need help. This enables you to have control over your emotions and, therefore, your overall health.

What is more is that they aren't just for emotional health. These techniques can be helpful for any problem, from eliminating a headache to taking 15 points off your golf score.

Once in awhile, I'd have a patient who expressed concerns about doing EFT because s/he did not know if the positive effects that occur with EFT were coming from God or from another source.

It is important to understand that energy therapies are not magical healing powers and are not coming from a source other than yourself. Your body has the capacity to heal itself when you remove the obstacles to cure. EFT is merely a tool to help you remove some of those obstacles.

There are many modalities of energy psychology available. You can learn more about Energy Psychology at www.energypsych.org. Of all the techniques out there, our favorite is Emotional Freedom Technique (EFT).

TAKE CONTROL

EFT Has Been The Biggest Help For Her

EFT has been by far the biggest help for me—I soon noticed immediate, incredible and lasting improvement. Since following the Take Control of Your Health program, I have more energy. My thyroid is in the normal range and I no longer see a doctor each week. By following the plan, I have become independently healthy!

—*Sherri Kaiser, Dacula, Georgia* ❧

Emotional Freedom Technique

EFT is a relatively recent innovation that was devised in the early '90s by Gary Craig. It has provided thousands with relief from pain, diseases and emotional issues. Simply stated, EFT involves tapping on acupuncture points while you tune into your problem. The process is easy to memorize and is portable so you can do it anywhere.

In order to clear your emotional baggage, Gary Craig suggests a protocol for optimal health called *The Personal Peace Procedure*. This procedure is to make a list of all the traumatic events that have occurred in your life, and, on a daily basis, use EFT on one of these events. This way you can begin to heal the negative events that may be stored in your energy system causing blockages to health and healing.

Clearing negative thoughts and emotions is one part of the healing process. The other part is learning new life skills that incorporate living by spiritual truths in a practical way so that you can continue to increase your state of well-being.

For a comprehensive listing of Energy Psychology and EFT Resources please go to mercola.com/eft

CHAPTER:

Sleep

Odds Are You Just Aren't Getting Enough Sleep.

According to the National Sleep Poll, the number of Americans getting more than 8 hours of sleep a night has dropped by 9% just since 1998, and the number of Americans getting less than 6 hours has gone up in that time from 12% to 16%. The reasons were pretty equally divided between having too many responsibilities to sleep and staying up to watch TV or to use the internet. Adolescents are also getting less sleep than they did a decade ago.[1]

Another study found that even when people believed that they got 7.5 hours of sleep, they actually averaged about 6.1 hours of sleep. Self-reported sleep is usually an underestimate. So whatever sleep you think you're getting, you're probably getting even less.

But What Are The Consequences Of This Loss Of Sleep On Your Health?

The American Cancer Society studied one million volunteers and found that there is an optimal amount of sleep for longevity, which seemed to be about 7 hours a night for adults.[2]

Perhaps because there is a tendency towards workaholism in the American culture (and also in other industrialized nations), it is likely difficult for you to put aside your responsibilities and make yourself go to bed on time to get enough sleep. Sleeping probably seems too lazy an activity for busy, responsible people such as yourself. Well, perhaps it is time to also put a sufficient number of hours of sleep on the "to do" list. The advantages of sleep can hardly be overstated, since sleep benefits most major organ systems and improves many markers of longevity. More to the point are the major diseases that sleep helps to prevent—such illnesses include cancer, diabetes, cardiovascular disease, and cognitive and memory decline, as well as accelerated aging.

TAKE CONTROL

Sounder Sleep and Forty Pound Weight Loss in the Frigid North

I reluctantly purchased Dr. Mercola's Take Control of Your Health Program thinking it can't work. Nothing else has. But you know what? It did! I lost 12 pounds the first month! And I'm down 40 pounds now. With every pound I lost, I gained a ton of energy in its place.

I wish my computer had the capability of sending a photo of myself to you. I'd like everyone to see what Dr. Mercola's help has done for me, with the advice on a healthy diet and supplements, good hydration, sound sleep, and the right kind of exercise. I'm 62, almost 63. Just imagine a tight, toned, young slim body, with radiant skin and a happy smile, that's me!

—*Jean Watts, Fairbanks, AK* ∾

A Good Night's Sleep Is Important For Your Immune System

Sleep deprivation weakens your immune system,[3] leaving you more susceptible to other diseases and disorders like, cancer and even the common cold. It is not uncommon for many people who suffer from sleep deprivation due to sleep disorders—sleep apnea, narcolepsy, insomnia, etc.—to also suffer from other problems, including diabetes, asthma, or a second sleep disorder.

Sleep deprivation also causes much stress and again, stress weakens our immune system—a double whammy. Both sleep deprivation and stress can upset your mental processes. You may suffer from confusion, memory loss, irritability, or emotional highs and lows. If you already have a mental disorder, sleep deprivation only adds to the problem.

Sleep Well Or Run The Risk Of Developing Heart Disease

One study, conducted on nurses, found that those who slept five hours or less per night had a 39% increase in cardiovascular disease.[4]

High blood pressure, clinically known as hypertension, is an early indicator of cardiovascular disease. Studies have shown that people who sleep for only four hours have a higher blood pressure and heart rate for eight hours after waking than subjects who were allowed a full eight hours of sleep.[5]

These findings suggest that your sympathetic nervous system—that is, your fight-or-flight mechanism that you use to cope with emergencies—becomes activated when you don't sleep enough. Later in this chapter, we'll review some ways to calm your sympathetic nervous system before you go to sleep.

Sleep Deficiency Can Actually Increase Your Risk Of Diabetes

Diabetes is another deadly disease that is more likely to strike those who do not get adequate sleep. A 2003 study followed 70,000 diabetes-free women for a period of 10 years and found that they had a 34% greater risk of developing diabetes than women who slept 7 or 8 hours a night.[6]

Studies of men have also shown almost *twice the risk* for diabetes among those sleeping 6 hours or less per night.[7] This is a serious issue, as one out of three people in the United States have either diabetes or pre-diabetes.

One reason for this is that sleep deprivation can result in a low glucose tolerance. Low glucose tolerance[8] means that there is not an optimal level of insulin released; insulin helps cells store glucose as energy, and a lack of it can result in hyperglycemia (high blood sugars) which can in turn, lead to diabetes.

Not Enough Sleep Can Make You Fat

It is now well-established that inadequate sleep is a factor in obesity. Fourteen different studies have found higher rates of obesity among people of all ages who reported getting inadequate sleep.[9]

The reason sleep deprivation causes weight gain is because it causes hormone disruption.[10] Sleep deprivation:

- Increases **cortisol**, which causes increased appetite and fat deposition around your mid-section. Memory loss and insulin resistance (a precursor to diabetes) can also result from an increase in cortisol.

- Increases **ghrelin**, which increases appetite and prevents the body from using up its excess fat stores.

- Decreases **leptin**, which causes the body to crave more food, especially carbohydrates.

- Decreases **insulin**, which increases the appetite, and leads to low blood sugar levels and insulin resistance.

Sleep Enough or Risk Being Depressed

Studies have shown that loss of sleep leads to a reduction in serotonin levels, which slowly over time, can lead to depression.[11]

Not Enough Sleep Impairs Your Thinking

Studies demonstrate that sleep-deprived hospital staff and residents make a significant number of serious medical errors, averaging 36% more than those with adequate sleep.[12]

If Growth Hormone is the Fountain of Youth, Then Sleep Is the Pump under the Fountain

Growth hormone has many functions, such as increasing the growth of children and promoting muscle mass in adults. It does this by increasing the number of new muscle cells.

Growth hormone promotes lipolysis, which is the breakdown of fats, resulting in a decrease of body fat. Growth hormone enhances the function and longevity of the beta cells of the pancreas, which are responsible for releasing insulin to help metabolize carbohydrates. Growth hormone also stimulates the immune system, to enable you to better protect yourself from infectious microbes. The two most powerful stimuli for the secretion of growth hormone are sleep and exercise. If you do not get enough sleep, you may become deficient in growth hormone.

Melatonin:

Why You Need Pitch Black Darkness All Night Long

Your bedroom should be so black at night that you can't even tell where the window is, so black that if you get up to use the bathroom during the night, you would have to grope your way forward slowly in order not to collide with anything. This may seem like an unrealistic suggestion, but if your drapes are heavy enough, you should be able to block out all outside light.

Hopefully, you don't live right next to flashing neon signs. If this is the case, you will need black-out shades or drapes as well. If you have a digital clock in your bedroom, turn it face down so the light does not show, as even this small amount of light can affect your sleep. Nightlights are out of the question for the bedroom.

If you simply are unable to make the investment to darken your sleeping room completely then you will want to consider an eye mask. I have used them when flying on planes overnight and they really do make a difference. However, it is definitely an inferior option to having a completely dark room while you are sleeping.

Once you get your bedroom totally dark, you have a strong, health-saving advantage for getting a good night's sleep. That advantage is melatonin.

Melatonin is a natural hormone produced by your pineal gland (a light-sensitive gland at the base of your brain) and is released when darkness falls. Melatonin makes you feel drowsy and helps you to achieve a deep and restful sleep. But melatonin does more than just help you sleep—it helps support your immune system function to support healing while you are asleep.

Optimal melatonin production is important for your health. Melatonin is produced by the pineal gland in a diurnal rhythm, but electric lights, which keep the room bright even after the sun sets, suppress melatonin production. As soon as you are faced with either the light of day or someone turning on a light in the middle of the night, your melatonin production suddenly shuts off, and it becomes harder to get back to sleep afterward. As a consequence, people who keep bright lights on until they go to bed at midnight only have optimal melatonin production for half of the 8–10 hours of sleep they should be getting.

Melatonin and Cancer

Melatonin is one of the strongest anti-oxidants and many experts believe it is one of the most important cancer-fighters.[13] In laboratory animals, the disruption of the body's natural daily rhythms has caused cancerous tumors to grow two to three times faster. Furthermore, melatonin has been found to slow the production of estrogen, which can promote certain types of cancer.

Recent research has shown that exposure to light at night significantly increases the risk of breast cancer. Three recent randomized control trials completed in Italy demonstrated that melatonin supplementation not only substantially decreased the side-effects associated with chemotherapy for advanced cancer (including metastatic breast cancer), but more than doubled response to chemotherapy and one-year survival rates.

Some of the cancer risk caused by disrupted sleep may also come from the resulting abnormal cortisol rhythms. Disrupted cortisol rhythms have been tied to a loss of natural-killer cells, which help your body fight cancer. Another hormone that is increased by inadequate sleep is insulin, and high levels of insulin are also linked to cancer.[14]

If you feel you need a good reason to get quality sleep, cancer prevention alone is an extremely worthy goal. Cancer, as everyone knows, is one of the most challenging diseases to treat. With cancer, prevention is by far your best option. It's time to seriously question and assess your late evening activities. Are they really so urgent or compelling that they are worth such a cancer risk as lack of sleep?

Melatonin And Your Brain

Melatonin also has important effects on your brain. People with seasonal affective disorder (SAD) have melatonin levels that fluctuate considerably during the year, whereas normal individuals have fairly stable melatonin throughout the year.[15]

Melatonin also benefits your memory. Researchers induced diabetes in rats, which inhibited their learning and memory. Then they dosed the rats with melatonin and Vitamin E, which significantly improved learning performance and memory. Both of these antioxidants help prevent the fats found in your brain from going rancid.[16]

Secrets To A Good Night's Sleep

Food And Drink To Avoid

- It is best to avoid eating before bedtime, especially grains and sugars. These simple carbohydrates break down to simple sugars and raise your blood sugar, which is stimulating and interferes with drifting off to sleep. Worse yet, simple carbs raise your blood sugar for a very short period. They then abruptly lower your blood sugar, leaving you hypoglycemic, which itself can awaken you and prevent your return to sleep.

- Also avoid alcohol. Although it makes people drowsy, that effect is of short duration, and you may wake up several hours later and feel that you cannot go back to sleep. Alcohol also keeps sleep light, which is not optimal for the repair and restorative functions that deep sleep accomplishes for you.

- If caffeine keeps you awake, try to avoid it in the afternoon. Caffeine is metabolized slowly by many people. Although some people can drink coffee and be ready for sleep an hour later, many others cannot sleep if they have had any afternoon caffeine. Amphetamine analogs, such as diet pills or the drugs used for ADHD (Ritalin, Adderall, Concerta, etc.), can promote wakefulness.

- If you know you are sensitive to certain foods, it would be best to avoid them. Delayed food sensitivity may appear one to three days after the ingested antigenic food. Dairy and wheat are very common culprits. For many people, they cause abdominal upset, gas, sinus congestion, and even sleep apnea.

- Don't drink any fluids within two to three hours of bedtime, so that before bed, you have the opportunity to void the liquids you have consumed during the day. That way, there is less chance of your sleep getting disturbed by the need to go to the bathroom.

Exercise

Exercise is the best natural sleep aid but only if done early in the day (morning is best), not near your bedtime. Exercise tires you out in all the right ways, and later when your body is ready to repair muscle tissue from your workouts, you will be ready for a sound sleep to enable that repair. Exercise for at least 20–30 minutes. Around five days a week is best, but you should try for at least three times per week. If you aren't already exercising, this is a great excuse to start your program now! Exercise includes aerobic (walking, biking, etc.) and anaerobic workouts (PACE, weights, sprints).

Energy and Light

As discussed above, it is important to sleep in complete darkness. Even the smallest amount of light can disrupt your daily rhythm of melatonin and serotonin levels and can shut off your production of these hormones for the rest of the night. Even if you go to the bathroom in the night, don't turn on the light. It is better to take a few more moments to walk and move slowly in the dark than to assault your eyes and brain with light while it is still in sleep mode.

Avoid Electromagnetic Fields (EMFs)

It would be best to eliminate all electricity from your bedroom. Even after you turn off the light, residual electricity is circulating through the wires in the walls, which has a mildly stimulating effect on your body. Dr. Herbert Ross, author of *Sleep Disorders*, goes so far as to recommend that you kill all power in the house by pulling your circuit breaker before going to bed.

If any electrical clock or other device must be in your bedroom, keep it at least three feet from your bed and pointed away from you, because of the EMFs they emit. Make sure your bedroom is not awash in electromagnetic fields. Like light, such fields disrupt the pacesetting of the pineal gland in managing melatonin and serotonin in the brain. You can measure EMFs with an inexpensive gaussmeter that can be easily found and purchased online.

Alarm Clocks

If you have a clock radio or other fluorescent alarm clock, then during periods of insomnia you may worry about the time and how you can't sleep, leading to a progressively worsening cycle. Therefore, it's best to turn the clock facedown at night.

Loud alarm clocks are also stressful for your body. If you are regularly getting enough sleep, you should not even need an alarm clock, because your body and mind adjust to your regular wake-up schedule. Sun alarm clocks or dawn simulators are excellent choices if you need to use an alarm clock They will not startle your adrenal system as traditional alarms do because they go on gradually and closely approximate a normal wake cycle by having the light gradually come on so you wake up more naturally.

Evening Activities That Will Prepare You For Bed

Get in the habit of going to bed early. Before the invention of electricity, our ancestors were in the habit of going to bed shortly after sundown. Being asleep by 9:00 p.m. in the winter and 10 p.m. in the summer gives your adrenal glands the opportunity to repair and recharge. During this time, your gallbladder also dumps toxins. So it is a good idea to keep your body rested and let these internal organs do the cleansing and repair they need to perform.

Also, don't change your bedtime. This just makes it harder for your pineal gland to adjust to the new schedule with appropriate levels of neurotransmitters and hormones. Once you get used to a certain sleep schedule, it is easier to get sleepy and then wake up at the usual times.

Often sleeplessness is due to the common condition of "busy brain." If you suffer from busy brain, you may be lying awake with many plans and other thoughts racing around your head. For this, you may find it helpful to keep a journal, so you can write down your thoughts before bed. This is a kind of catharsis which allows you to release your thoughts so they don't haunt you through the night.

Read something calming, spiritual, or religious in order to help you to relax. Don't read stimulating material, such as crime stories or suspense novels, because if it is a page-turner of a good story, you might end up turning those pages all night long.

Many people feel more relaxed listening to relaxation CD's of music, nature sounds such as a waterfall or the ocean, white noise, or brainwave-enhancing audio technology. Keep your bed for sleeping. If you are in the habit of eating or doing work or crossword puzzles, or watching TV in bed, then you are associating stimulating activity with a place that should be used just for sleeping. It is the wrong association. Reserve your bed for sleep.

Television can ruin your health in multiple ways. The U.S. Census Bureau in 2007 documented that the average person in the United States watches 4.5 hours of TV **every day**. While I firmly believe you need to significantly reduce this amount in general, you clearly don't need any TV exposure prior to bed. The fast-moving images and routine over dramatization are too stimulating to the brain, as you need to wind down for the evening. The flickering lights and colors are too stimulating to the pineal gland that needs to prepare for sleep.

Health And Wellness Considerations

If you are overweight, work towards achieving a normal body weight. Being overweight is a risk for sleep apnea, which is a condition where a person frequently stops breathing during sleep and awakens throughout the night to restart the breathing process. Sleep apnea prevents a restful night's sleep.

Insomnia can also be caused by excessive levels of the hormone cortisol.[17] This may reflect a dysfunction of the hypothalamic-pituitary-adrenal axis, which is just a fancy way of saying that your brain may be telling the adrenal glands to pump out too much cortisol. On the other hand, it could be the adrenal function itself which needs treatment.

Menopausal and perimenopausal women may have insomnia as a result of fluctuating hormones, resulting in hot flashes or other stimulus for night-time waking. If you suspect any of the above conditions, check with a physician specializing in natural medicine (such as a naturopathic doctor) for diagnosis and treatment. Also note, that many over-the-counter and prescription drugs can affect your sleep so be sure and check your medications for side-effects.

Temperature Considerations

If you have cold feet, try wearing socks to bed. Feet have the most sluggish circulation in your body, so they often feel cold before the rest of the body does. One study has shown that people who wore socks to bed had the least nighttime waking.[18] What a great simple, non-toxic, no-cost way to enhance your sleep!

However, your bedroom should not be too hot. Keep the temperature in your bedroom 60–70 degrees F, at least in cool weather.

Another way of relaxing is to take a hot bath, shower, or sauna before bed. When body temperature is raised in the late evening, it will fall again at bedtime, and this cooling promotes sleepiness.

Supplements

Homeopathy, meaning "like cures like," is an energetic system of medicine that matches the symptoms of an energetic remedy to the symptoms that the person has, and these symptoms cancel each other out. Homeopathy is very individualized, but one of the more common remedies given for insomnia is the homeopathic remedy of coffee (homeopathic remedies are diluted so many times, there is no physical substance of coffee in the remedy). If homeopathic coffee doesn't work, consider getting a consultation with a trained homeopath or naturopathic doctor.

As a last resort, you can supplement with sublingual tablets or drops of melatonin 0.05–0.5 mg 1–30 minutes before bedtime. However, these tablets should be used with caution. Some people have reported vivid dreams or nightmares with melatonin use. Your best option is to increase melatonin with full spectrum fluorescent bulbs in winter and exposure to bright sunlight, preferably an hour per day, during good weather, as well as complete darkness at night as previously described.

You can also use L-tryptophan or 5-HTP as a precursor to melatonin. L-tryptophan is safer than straight melatonin. It is simply an amino acid, and it is common in many foods. However, to get enough tryptophan from food sources to make a difference in your sleep, you would have to eat massive amounts of food.

Tryptophan and 5-HTP have been found to be helpful with insomnia. Tryptophan has been helpful for reducing sleep latency (the length of time it takes to fall asleep.)[19] This has proven true over numerous studies for people with insomnia, people with normal sleep patterns, and in animal studies. Tryptophan also does not produce distortions of sleep physiology when first administered, during long-term use, or after withdrawal. Unlike the pharmaceutical sedatives and hypnotics, tryptophan is a molecule that is actually a natural part of our bodies and the food we eat.

5-HTP, which is 5-hydroxytryptophan, has been found to be of benefit for children's nightmares, according to a study in which almost all of the children who took 5-HTP improved their night-mares and almost all of the children given placebos did not.[20]

Other Helpful Considerations to Help You Sleep Better:

- Establish a bedtime routine (this could include deep breathing, meditation, aromatherapy/essential oils, massage, etc.)

- Go to the bathroom right before bed so you will reduce the chance you'll wake up to go in the middle of the night)

- Put work away at least an hour or two before bed so your mind has a chance to relax

Sleep Labs

If you have tried everything and you still aren't sleeping, or never feel rested, you may consider seeing a sleep lab, especially if you are significantly overweight. Many people have discovered that they have sleep apnea and have benefited from a CPAP machine while they worked on losing weight.

At any rate, be sure to make a good night's sleep one of your top priorities. Your body deserves it.

TAKE CONTROL

Her Sleep and Her Whole Life Started to Turn Around

I'd like to share with you the story I received from *Anna Wyatt in Wells, ME* ⮞

For many months, the morning sunlight was creeping into my room far too early for my taste. It seemed as if each night, my exhausted body would collapse into bed and after struggling to fall asleep for far too long, would eventually drift into a fitful few hours before that sun noiselessly splashed across my face, waking me with a silence that was still too loud to me.

Another day as an exhausted, overworked, over-stressed, single mom would await me and inwardly, I'd groan. I was not sleeping well, I was not waking well, and I simply was not functioning well. During the week, the mercola.com newsletter would pop into my e-mail box and I'd usually take a few seconds to glance over the text and see if anything really caught my eye. For the most part, that's where I stopped.

Then I got sick. It wasn't just a little cold and it didn't go away in the 3 days I had hoped for. Days turned into weeks, and those weeks spilled over into a month. This was just unacceptable. I needed to be well, I couldn't afford to take time off and my kids didn't have their mom at her best. I deserved better, they deserved better. I needed to step it up.

But finally, it occurred to me that if I took just one article a week and tried to apply it to my life, within a very short amount of time; I'd have made more than a handful of significant changes. And I knew that these changes would only be for the better. So I started with just one change from an article I read in mercola.com and suddenly, I started to feel better. I incorporated a few changes into my diet. Suddenly, my energy came back and my sleep started to improve.

From there I ordered Dr. Mercola's Take Control of Your Health Program and am pouring through it like there's no tomorrow. I cannot wait to apply even more changes to my previously energy-starved life. I will benefit, my children will benefit, and I'm already spreading the news to those near and dear to me. My quest for health has begun and I'm so excited.

CHAPTER:

Artificial Sweeteners

You see the little packets of artificial sweeteners laid out for you whenever you go to a restaurant. There they are in pink, blue, and yellow—the colors of baby clothes. They're in all your diet sodas and snacks. But still, there's a nagging question at the back of your mind when you see them. *Are these really safe?*

You are right to ask that question. The answer is no.

Artificial sweeteners are just about the worst of all possible worlds, as far as dietary choices go: they are completely unnatural, insufficiently tested for safety, unnecessary in the diet, and have a long history of causing health problems. They are powerful examples of a diet gone mad.

I cover this topic in much greater detail in my 2006 book, *Sweet Deception* (SweetDeception.com), but this chapter should help to give you a good idea of why artificial sweeteners are so harmful to your health; it will also touch on some of the shocking collusions between government and big business which have allowed these dangerous chemicals to become part of the human diet.

What Are Artificial Sweeteners Anyway?

"Artificial" means something that is not found in nature, but is instead a man-made chemical compound. Artificial sweeteners do not contain nutrients like vitamins and minerals, and they are very low in carbohydrates and calories. The world consumption of artificial sweeteners now stands at 7.5 million metric tons per year, including annual sales of over four billion gallons of diet soda.

Current artificial sweeteners include (in order of creation):

- Saccharin
- Cyclamate
- Aspartame
- Acesulfame-K
- Sucralose
- Alitame
- Neotame

My position on all artificial sweeteners is that you should simply avoid them: I believe that you should stick to the food your body was designed to eat, ideally foods as they are found in their unprocessed state in nature.

Saccharin

In 1879, Dr. Ira Remsen, a well-known chemist, and Constantine Fahlberg, a research fellow, were experimenting with toluene derivatives at Johns Hopkins University. Toluene is a clear, colorless, and hazardous chemical produced in the process of making gasoline from crude oil.

One of these two scientists made a serendipitous discovery, using a method that would eventually become the standard procedure for creating an artificial sweetener: accidentally spilling and then ingesting chemicals. In this particular case, the researcher spilled a toluene derivative onto his hand, and later that evening he noticed his food at dinner tasted oddly sweet. He traced the taste back to the chemicals, and named the substance saccharin, after the word *saccharide*, which means complex sugar.[1]

Which man made the discovery? Well, according to Remsen, it was Remsen—but according to Fahlberg, it was Fahlberg. Whichever one it was, in 1884 Fahlberg patented saccharin and began mass-producing it—without crediting Remsen, Johns Hopkins University, or anyone else. Fahlberg became fabulously wealthy, and Remsen did not. "Fahlberg is a scoundrel," Remsen later commented. "It nauseates me to hear my name mentioned in the same breath with him."[2]

The illustrious history of the marketing of artificial sweeteners had begun.

Saccharin contains only one-eighth of a calorie per teaspoon and is approximately three hundred times sweeter than sugar. It was introduced to the marketplace with great success both in the United States and in Europe. In 1901, a company called Monsanto was formed for the sole purpose of producing saccharin. By 1903, Monsanto began producing saccharin for an obscure new company called Coca-Cola. And in 1912, saccharin was banned as a result of public concerns about possible health risks. But the ban didn't last very long. In 1914, the sugar rationing of World War I created a demand for artificial sweeteners, and health concerns were brushed aside in the face of economic ones. The Second World War had a similar effect, and by 1945 saccharin use was commonplace.[3]

Saccharin created the foundation for sugar-free products worldwide and is still used in tabletop sweeteners, toothpaste, baked goods, chewing gum, candy, dessert toppings, mouthwash, and many other products.

Saccharin's potential health risks were not examined thoroughly until many decades later, as a result of the next artificial sweetener to achieve widespread popularity.

Cyclamate

In 1937, University of Illinois graduate student Michael Sveda discovered cyclamate in a manner astonishingly similar to the method used to find saccharin. Sveda was trying to synthesize fever-reducing drugs and laid the cigarette he was smoking down on a lab bench. When he placed it in his mouth again, he discovered the sweet taste of cyclamate from the experimental drugs he had on his fingers.

Cyclamate had less aftertaste than saccharin, and its discovery led to the introduction, in 1957, of the first artificial sweetener blend— Sweet'N Low®. Sweet'N Low was originally a mixture of cyclamate and saccharin; the mixture masked the off-taste of each sweetener. Sweet'N Low was the first artificial sweetening agent to be marketed in powdered form, imitating the appearance, texture, and taste of sugar.

It was a tremendous commercial success, and to this day, little pink packets of Sweet'N Low are a familiar sight at restaurants and coffee shops across the United States. Along with Sweet'N Low, diet drinks such as Diet Rite and Tab were also introduced, using the same cyclamate/saccharin blend with great financial success.

Both saccharin and cyclamate were introduced before the 1958 Food Additives Amendment to the Food, Drug, and Cosmetic Act, and were therefore automatically classified in the Generally Recognized As Safe (GRAS) food additive category when the act was passed, meaning neither was required to be thoroughly tested for safety.

But in 1969, cyclamate was banned by the FDA. Some research studies seemed to indicate that cyclamate caused cancer in laboratory mice.[4] One part of the 1958 Food Additives Amendment, the Delaney Clause, sets a zero tolerance for any chemical found to cause cancer in animal testing. But many thought the studies were questionable, and cyclamate continues to be used in more than fifty-five countries, including the British Commonwealth.

Sweet'N Low is currently a mixture of saccharin and dextrose.

"Saccharin Has Been Determined to Cause Cancer in Laboratory Animals"

The concern over cyclamate soon resulted in saccharin being tested for safety for the very first time—nearly one hundred years after its introduction into the human diet. In the late 1970s, a scientist named Douglas Arnold performed a study finding that saccharin caused bladder cancer in laboratory animals (although this has not been shown in humans). Additional studies confirmed the increased risk of bladder tumors in animals.[5-7]

The Canadian government immediately outlawed saccharin. The FDA proposed to likewise ban the sweetener but was met by a great deal of public opposition; after the cyclamate ban, saccharin was the only artificial sweetener available for general use. Congress intervened and allowed saccharin to be sold as long as the products containing it carried a warning label reading: "Use of this product may be hazardous to your health. This product contains saccharin, which has been determined to cause cancer in laboratory animals."[8]

In 1991, long-term studies did demonstrate some correlation between saccharin use and cancer, but not enough for saccharin to be considered a "major" cancer risk factor. In 1992, tests performed on rats showed that they had physiological differences from humans that made them more susceptible to bladder cancer from saccharin. So, in 2000, President Clinton signed into law that cancer warnings were no longer required for saccharin products.[9]

Somewhat ironically, considering its reputation, saccharin is probably the safest artificial sweetener on the market. But considering that it is derived from toluene, and does raise your risk of cancer to some degree, I believe even it should be avoided.

Aspartame

Aspartame was originally developed in a laboratory as a drug to treat peptic ulcer disease. In 1965, James Schlatter, a scientist at G. D. Searle & Company, licked his fingers to pick up a piece of paper, and got the world's first taste of this chemical.

You may recognize aspartame by its other names: NutraSweet and Equal. Equal is more easily recognized as the little blue packets found on nearly every restaurant table in the United States. NutraSweet is sold in over one hundred countries, found in over six thousand products, and is consumed by over 250 million people. Aspartame dominated the industry until Splenda came along in the late nineties.

H. J. Roberts, MD, coined the term "aspartame disease" to encompass the symptoms and public health implications relating to this chemical sweetener.[10] There have been more reports to the FDA for aspartame reactions than all other food additives combined (with the exception of Olestra®). Dr. Roberts states that by 1988, *80 percent of complaints to the FDA about food additives* had to deal with aspartame products.[11] Aspartame is undoubtedly one of the most controversial food additives in modern times.

Aspartame was the first artificial sweetener to be developed after the 1958 amendments requiring pre-market proof of safety. Early safety studies of aspartame identified potential neurotoxic side effects. In one study, five out of seven monkeys fed aspartame had grand mal seizures, and a sixth died. Research conducted by neuroscientist Dr. John Olney showed that aspartic acid, one of the main ingredients in aspartame, caused damage to the brains of infant mice. Searle's own scientists confirmed these findings in similar studies.[12]

Corporate leaders at G. D. Searle, nonetheless, invested tens of millions of dollars into conducting tests geared towards winning aspartame's approval by the FDA.

Aspartame Causes First Ever FDA-Initiated Criminal Investigation

In 1977, the FDA requested that the U.S. attorney's office investigate Searle for alleged inaccuracies and inadequate testing procedures and for misrepresenting their findings[13]—the first time in history that the FDA requested a criminal investigation of a food manufacturer. The probe into Searle's activities uncovered many problems with their testing procedures.[14,15]

In March of 1977, political powerhouse Donald Rumsfeld, who would later become U.S. secretary of defense under George W. Bush, joined G. D. Searle as their new CEO.[16] Soon after, the law firm that represented Searle began contract negotiations with Samuel Skinner—the U.S. attorney leading the investigation against Searle. In July 1977, Skinner left the U.S. attorney's office and took a position with Searle's law firm, Sidley & Austin. Skinner's sudden resignation stalled the grand jury investigation for long enough that the statute of limitations ran out, forcing the grand jury to abandon its investigation.

In August of 1977, the FDA released the Bressler Report, by Dr. Jerome Bressler, which identified additional errors and inconsistent findings in the aspartame safety studies. The Bressler Report found, among other problems, that Searle had reported obvious tumors as normal—in one case malignant lymphoma was recorded as being "normal lymphatic swelling."[17]

In 1979, the FDA established a Public Board of Inquiry (PBOI) to rule on safety issues surrounding NutraSweet, and within one year, concluded that aspartame should not be approved pending further investigations of brain tumors in animals.

Donald Rumsfeld Gets Aspartame Approved

In 1981, Rumsfeld's political ally, Ronald Reagan, became the fortieth president of the United States. Rumsfeld reportedly made a commitment to getting aspartame approved within a year.[18]

Within one month, Reagan replaced the FDA commissioner with his puppet, Dr. Arthur Hull Hayes.[19] Dr. Hayes appointed an internal panel to review the issues raised by the FDA Public Board of Inquiry. After the panel ruled three-to-two to uphold the ban on aspartame, Dr. Hayes installed a sixth member who tied the vote, which allowed him to cast another vote to break the tie and approve aspartame.[20]

Dr. Hayes, who had virtually no background in food additives, later took a job with G. D. Searle's public relations firm as a senior scientific consultant and was reportedly paid $1,000 a day.[21,22]

Why Is Aspartame So Potentially Toxic?

Aspartame has three components: phenylalanine, aspartic acid, and methyl ester.[23] Those who defend aspartame state that these substances are a harmless and natural part of our diet.

This, of course, is only a partial truth.

Aspartic acid is an amino acid that is normally supplied by the foods we eat; however, it can only be considered natural and harmless when it is consumed in combination with protein, fat, and carbohydrates in the form of genuine whole foods. When aspartic acid is consumed as a free-form amino acid, it enters your central nervous system in abnormally high concentrations, causing excessive firing of brain neurons and potential cell death. This effect has been termed *excitotoxicity*. It is linked to symptoms such as headaches, depression, mental confusion, balance problems, and seizures.[24-26]

Excitotoxicity was first observed by Dr. John Olney, who showed that a single dose of monosodium glutamate (MSG) could raise blood glutamate levels to the point of causing brain damage in the hypothalamus.[27] Olney's early scientific efforts led the baby food industry to remove MSG from all of their products. Olney later demonstrated that the aspartic acid in aspartame has the same effect as the very similar glutamic acid in MSG.

Today, the concept of free-form amino acids acting as excitotoxins is universally accepted. The scientific community has even embraced the potential of excitotoxicity to lead to the development of diseases such as Parkinson's and Alzheimer's. However, the FDA still refuses to recognize the danger. To date, they have not required any food manufacturers to remove potential excitotoxic amino acids from the food supply—MSG, aspartic acid, or any others.

Dr. H. J. Roberts, the foremost medical authority on aspartame, said that he has had many patients in their thirties and forties consult with him for symptoms of Alzheimer's. They were confused, forgetful, couldn't think. Once they stopped using aspartame, their symptoms disappeared.[28]

Aspartame Causes Mental Retardation In Phenylketonuria (PKU)

Phenylalanine is commonly known in association with the genetic disease phenylketonuria (PKU). PKU is characterized by the inability of the body to utilize phenylalanine, which causes a toxic buildup in the body that can lead to mental retardation unless proper care is taken. PKU is routinely screened for at birth.

People with PKU cannot, under any circumstance, eat any food containing phenylalanine, including aspartame. The FDA has therefore required the manufacturers of aspartame to put warning labels on all of their products to protect consumers.

Methanol

Even more worrisome is the 10 percent of aspartame that is absorbed into your bloodstream as methanol (aka wood alcohol, paint remover), a breakdown product of the methyl ester component. The EPA defines safe consumption of methanol as no more than 7.8 milligrams per day; a can of diet soda contains almost 16 milligrams of methanol. Methanol poisoning can result in fatal kidney damage, blindness, multiple organ system failure, and death.[29]

The manufacturers of aspartame defend the methanol produced in it by claiming it is found naturally in many foods. But in other foods, such as fruit and fruit juices, methanol is bound to pectin, which is a form of fiber. As a result of this bond, your body is not exposed to methanol, nor does it break it down. In fact, according to Dr. James Bowen, this quality of pectin is so well known that when professionals such as mechanics accidentally ingest methanol, they "will often successfully treat themselves by merely ingesting orange juice and going on about their work with no further problems."[30]

In aspartame, the methanol is not bound to pectin and is metabolized by your body.

DKP And Formaldehyde

Phenylalanine decomposes into DKP, a known carcinogen, when it is exposed to warm temperatures or prolonged storage. And even at cold temperatures, methanol can spontaneously break down to a colorless toxin known as formaldehyde.[31] Studies on formaldehyde exposure have shown side effects such as:

- Irreversible genetic damage (Shaham 1996)
- Headaches, fatigue, chest tightness (Main 1983)
- Sleeping problems, burning skin, fatigue, chest pain, dizziness (Liu 1991)
- Musculoskeletal, gastrointestinal, and cardiovascular symptoms (Srivastava 1992)
- Headaches, dizziness, nausea, lack of concentration ability (Burdach 1980)
- Cognitive adverse effects (Kilburn 2000)
- Seizures and neurobehavioral impairment (Kilburn 1994)
- Headaches, skin problems (Proietti 2002)
- Memory problems, equilibrium and dexterity impairment (Kilburn 1987)[32]

According to the EPA, formaldehyde can cause cancer in laboratory animals and likely causes cancer in humans.

Aspartame and Cancer

In January of 1984, one year after aspartame was approved for use in diet sodas, brain cancer rates began to skyrocket at a faster rate than any other form of cancer. This was happening at the same time that many other types of cancers were beginning to decrease in incidence. There has also been an increased occurrence of cancer in the brain and spinal cord among children whose mothers consumed aspartame throughout their pregnancy.[33,34]

In a study of 320 rats, twelve rats developed malignant brain tumors after receiving aspartame-containing feed for two years.[35] Recently, Dr. Morando Soffritti, a cancer researcher in Italy, performed an animal study that found aspartame was associated with an unusually high rate of leukemias and lymphomas.[36]

At Least One Million May Have Had Side Effects from Aspartame

The FDA has received over ten thousand complaints submitted by people who have had a reaction to aspartame. By the FDA's own admission, less than 1 percent of those who experience a reaction to a product ever report it. This means roughly a million people are a likely to have experienced reactions to aspartame.[37]

The reported symptoms have included migraines, aggressive behavior, depression, disorientation, hyperactivity, extreme numbness, excitability, memory loss, loss of depth perception, liver impairment, cardiac arrest, seizures, vision problems, suicidal tendencies, severe mood swings, and death.[38,39]

Many victims are not aware that aspartame may be at the root of their problems and end up spending a tremendous amount of time and money trying to figure out why they are sick.

Acesulfame-K

Acesulfame-K (also known under the brand name Sunett) was discovered in 1967 when chemist Karl Clauss, of the Hoechst AG Company, accidentally spilled some on his finger, which he then licked as he reached for a piece of paper.

Acesulfame-K was first approved for limited use by the FDA in July 1988 although it had been used in Europe starting five years before that. In the mid-1990s, Hoechst petitioned the FDA for acesulfame-K to be approved for use in soft drinks, which would greatly increase consumer exposure. It was at this point that concerned scientists raised objections. They asserted that the studies on which the sweetener's existing approval was based were seriously flawed, and that wider approval would lead to a public danger.

The nonprofit Center for Science in the Public Interest (CSPI) has repeatedly expressed concern that acesulfame-K is a potential carcinogen.[40] Acesulfame-K may contain methylene chloride, which can cause, after chronic exposure, headaches, mental confusion, depression, liver effects, kidney effects, bronchitis, loss of appetite, nausea, lack of balance, visual disturbances, and cancer.[41]

Scientific opposition to acesulfame-K has been ignored. In 1998, acesulfame-K was additionally approved for use in beverages. More recently, the FDA increased consumer exposure further by approving it for even broader use.

Splenda

Splenda is the trade name of an artificial sweetener that has pulled off one of the most successful consumer product launches in history. Between 2000 and 2004, the percentage of U.S. households using Splenda products jumped from 3 percent to 20 percent.[42] In 2005 retail sales of Splenda topped $187 million. 2005 retail sales were only $57 million for aspartame-based Equal and $51 million for saccharin-based Sweet'N Low.[43]

Part of the reason for Splenda's success is that it doesn't have the bitter metallic aftertaste of other artificial sweeteners. In addition, many manufacturers are abandoning the use of aspartame because of the health concerns and controversy surrounding it.

Splenda is the brand name for sucralose, a chlorinated artificial sugar derivative up to six hundred times sweeter than sugar. You, as a consumer, cannot buy sucralose by itself, as it is only available to manufacturers in quantities of no less than one kilogram, at a cost of over $450/kilogram. Splenda products, which are the versions available to consumers, consist of sucralose combined with other caloric sweeteners so that they measure and pour just like sugar.

Sucralose—A Serendipitous Surprise

In 1975, Shashikant Phadnis, an Indian graduate student in the chemistry department of Queen Elizabeth College in London, was working with his advisor, Leslie Hough, in their chemistry lab. They were trying to create new *insecticides*. The experiment involved taking sulfuryl chloride—a highly poisonous chemical—and adding it drop by drop to a sugar solution.

At one point in the procedure, Hough asked Phadnis to *test* the powder, but Phadnis thought Hough was telling him to *taste* it. He told Hough that it was sweet.

"When I reported my findings to Les, he asked if I was *crazy* . . . how could I taste compounds without knowing anything about their toxicity?" However, not long after, Hough was so excited about their discovery, he added some to his coffee. It was Phadnis this time who warned Hough about the unknown toxicity. "Oh, forget it," Hough replied, "We'll survive!"[44]

Hough and Phadnis teamed up with a British sugar company, Tate & Lyle, to experiment on hundreds of chlorinated sugars before they finally selected one. Substituting three chlorine ions for three hydroxyl groups on a sugar molecule resulted in the artificial chemical whose name is "1,6-dichloro-1,6-dideoxy-beta-D-fructofuranosyl-4-chloro-4-deoxy-alpha-D-galactopyranoside."[45] We can only assume this molecule was then renamed "sucralose" to make it sound more natural.

In 1980, Tate & Lyle sold the manufacturing rights of sucralose to Johnson & Johnson, one of the world's largest healthcare and pharmaceutical companies. Johnson & Johnson created a new company (McNeil Nutritionals LLC) to be solely responsible for Splenda marketing and production. Currently, McNeil is responsible for the marketing of Splenda brand products, and Tate & Lyle is responsible for manufacturing sucralose.[46]

How Sucralose Was Introduced Into The United States

Canada became the first country to approve the use of sucralose in 1991. In the United States, sucralose was denied approval by the FDA for eleven years (1987–1998).[47] Insiders say the delay occurred because other artificial sweetener companies didn't want the competition and prevented it from being approved. Sucralose was suddenly approved around the same time Monsanto was asking for FDA approval of aspartame's chemical cousin, neotame. The competition stopped protesting the approval of sucralose for fear that McNeil would try to sabotage the approval of neotame.[48]

In any case, with no warning, the FDA suddenly approved sucralose on April 1, 1998. McNeil was caught off-guard by the sudden approval and had to scramble to build a facility that could meet the demand.[49]

The Sucralose Studies

To research sucralose, I carefully plodded through the two-foot stack of documents and memorandums that were involved in the FDA final ruling for the approval of sucralose as a food additive.

> "Something is seriously wrong here."

There are only six published human studies on sucralose. The longest sucralose was studied in the published human trials was thirteen weeks. McNeil did submit unpublished research to the FDA that studied humans taking sucralose for a total of six months, but these studies only focused on the effect of sucralose on blood sugar in diabetics.

Out of eighty-four published studies, only ten were animal studies designed to evaluate the safety of sucralose. We are aware of only three long-term trials in animals: one study using 104 mice,[50] one using 104 rats over a two year period, and a twelve-month oral toxicity study in dogs.[51]

After carefully reviewing the evidence, I have concluded that there are simply no long-term safety trials done on any humans, none, nada, zero, zip, not one to assure you that using this sweetener for years will not cause you serious health problems.

Something is seriously wrong here.

"Made From Sugar, So It Tastes Like Sugar"

McNeil Nutritionals has gone to great lengths to suggest that Splenda is natural and safe by using the slogan, "Made from sugar, so it tastes like sugar." But after the lengthy chemical transformation process it goes through, it is anything but a sugar molecule:[52]

1. Sucrose is tritylated with trityl chloride in the presence of dimethylformamide and 4-methylmorpholine, and the tritylated sucrose is then acetylated with acetic anhydride.

2. The resulting sucrose molecule TRISPA (6,1',6'-tri-O-tritylpenta-O acetylsucrose) is chlorinated with hydrogen chlorine in the presence of toluene.

3. The resulting 4-PAS (sucrose 2,3,4,3',4'-pentaacetate) is heated in the presence of methyl isobutyl ketone and acetic acid.

4. The resulting 6-PAS (sucrose 2,3,6,3',4'-pentaacetate) is chlorinated with thionyl chloride in the presence of toluene and benzyltriethlyammonium chloride.

5. The resulting TOSPA (sucralose pentaacetate) is treated with methanol in the presence of sodium methoxide to produce sucralose.

Nowhere in nature is there any form of sugar that remotely resembles the resulting chlorinated hydrocarbon known as sucralose. This product is not natural, nor is it a real sugar. It isn't even close.

What You Need to Know About the Chlorine in Sucralose

Chlorine is a chemical element, and according to the EPA, a class-one carcinogen (cancer-causing agent).[53] According to McNeil's Web site, Splenda.com, we shouldn't worry about the chlorine in sucralose, as it is already a part of our food supply, present naturally in many foods and beverages, such as salt.[54] But the chlorine in Splenda is completely different from the chloride in salt. In salt, there is a stable bond between the chlorine and sodium. In Splenda, the chlorine atoms are instead bonded with carbon.

Molecules which contain bonds between chlorine and carbons are called *chlorocarbons* or *organochlorines*. As Dr. James Bowen, a physician and biochemist, writes, the bond between chlorine and carbon makes chlorocarbons harmful to life:

> Unlike sodium chloride, chlorocarbons are never nutritionally compatible with our metabolic processes and are wholly incompatible with normal human metabolic functioning . . . [C]hlorocarbons such as sucralose deliver chlorine directly into our cells through normal metabolization. This makes them effective insecticides . . .[55]

Organochlorines as a group are mainly used as pesticides, such as DDT, dieldrin, aldrin, lindane, chlordane, and heptachlor. Organochlorines have come under considerable scrutiny because of their persistence in the environment and the human body. Notorious organochlorines include "Agent Orange," and polychlorinated biphenyls (PCBs), which have consistently been associated with cancer and abnormalities within the reproductive, immune, and nervous systems.

Metabolism Of Sucralose

Normally, when you ingest an organochlorine, it is absorbed through your colon and enters your bloodstream, and your liver then attempts to detoxify it. If your detoxification mechanisms are overwhelmed by a high toxic load, your body will not be able to effectively eliminate organochlorines, and you will store them in your fat cells.

Organochlorines are fat-soluble by definition although their solubility can vary considerably. Fat-soluble substances tend to accumulate in organ tissues that are high in fat, such as your brain. And even worse—they are permanently stored there.[56]

McNeil strongly insists that sucralose is different from all the other organochlorines and is safely excreted from the body mostly unchanged. They claim that very little sucralose is absorbed into your bloodstream—although "very little" is not at all the same as "none". The Health Professionals section of Splenda.com states that approximately 15 percent of ingested sucralose is absorbed.[57] However, even that 15 percent number is an imprecise "average" absorption rate, based primarily on widely varying animal studies. The range for humans has been estimated to be 11–27 percent according to the FDA review of studies.

The FDA final ruling on sucralose concluded that sucralose is "poorly absorbed" following ingestion. An absorption rate of 27 percent is not what I call "poorly absorbed." That is almost one-third.

McNeil also claims that sucralose is somehow the exception to the organochlorine rule and is "almost insoluble in fat" (note the word "almost," which means that there is at least some fat solubility), and so will not be stored forever in your body. But even if this is the case, organochlorines don't have to be fat soluble to cause harm.

Splenda Metabolites

The FDA has stated that there may be at least twenty-one possible metabolites (digestion products) of sucralose.[58] Studies show that some of the metabolites of sucralose (such as 1,6-dichloro-1,6-dideoxyfructose—also known as 1,6-DCF) can cause:[59]

- Liver toxicity
- Weak mutagenic activity
- Enlarged livers in rat fetuses
- Low-birth weight in rat offspring
- Maternal and fetal toxicity

There are further reports of 1.6-DCF converting to a molecule called 6-chlorofructose, which caused paralysis in mice after only eight days of treatment.[60]

McNeil's position is that the FDA Final Rule states that the "no-observed effect" level for the metabolites is tens of thousands of times higher than the estimated daily intake (EDI) and, therefore, allows an adequate safety margin.

Interestingly, the FDA in its final ruling stated the available pharmacokinetic data *did not allow them to draw definitive conclusions regarding the bioaccumulations of sucralose and its breakdown products.* The FDA did argue that sucralose's low fat solubility, along with animal studies showing limited direct tissue toxicity and no evidence of cancer-causing activity in the breakdown products, eliminated any cause for concern.

I disagree with the FDA's conclusion; the vast majority of sucralose safety research was done on rats. Rats only absorb an average of 5 percent of ingested sucralose while humans have absorbed as much as 27 percent. Rats are not an exact model from which to base conclusions, and the differences could be critical.

Reported Side Effects From Sucralose

Hundreds of people have written letters describing the horrific symptoms they experienced after consuming sucralose. The following list contains some of the most common symptoms listed in the sucralose testimonials on Mercola.com:

- Skin—Redness, itching, swelling, blistering, weeping, crusting, rash, eruptions, or hives (itchy bumps or welts).

- Lungs—Wheezing, tightness, cough, or shortness of breath

- Head—Dry mouth and sinuses; swelling or inflammation of the face, eyelids, lips, tongue, or throat; headaches and migraines

- Nose—Stuffy nose, runny nose, sneezing

- Eyes—Red (bloodshot), itchy, swollen, or watery

- Stomach—Bloating, gas, pain, constipation, nausea, vomiting, diarrhea, or bloody diarrhea

- Heart—Chest pains, palpitations, or fluttering

- Joints—Joint pains or aches

- Neurological—Seizures, anxiety, anger, panic, insomnia, dizziness, spaced-out sensation, mood swings, depression

- Other—Bleeding readily without clotting, blood in urine, menstrual delay or missed period, night sweats, numbness of the limbs

Avoid The Deception

With Splenda, you are faced with an issue of deceptive advertising. As Michael Jacobson, the executive director of the Center for Science in the Public Interest, states, "'Made from sugar' certainly sounds better than, say, 'Made from chlorinated hydrocarbons,' 'Made in a laboratory,' or 'Fresh from the factory!'"[61]

According to pharmaceutical chemist Shane Ellison: "To use an organochlorine to make a sweetener defies logic. It is the first organochlorine ever used for human consumption. I would no sooner eat Splenda® than I would eat DDT."

Alitame

Alitame was developed by Pfizer Inc. in 1979. It is a white crystalline powder with a faint alcohol odor and is a closely related cousin of aspartame, sharing many of its characteristics. Alitame is already approved for use in a variety of food and beverage products in New Zealand, Mexico, Australia, and China, but its approval in the U.S. has been delayed pending a request by the FDA that Pfizer repeat a questionable animal study.

For the time being, little is known about alitame. Advocates for its approval describe one of its main assets as being its synergistic sweetening effect when combined with other low-calorie sweeteners. It would seem prudent, if the goal is to use alitame as a synergistic sweetener, that it be tested for safety in combination with other artificial sweeteners, but this is unlikely to happen.

Neotame

As the patent for aspartame was running out, Monsanto developed a new version of aspartame called neotame that is seventy-two times sweeter. Neotame was approved in 1997 for tabletop sweetener use, and in 2002 as a general-use sweetener. Sales of neotame increased by 400 percent from 2004 to 2005.[62]

The sweetest artificial sweetener ever invented, neotame is seven to thirteen thousand times sweeter than sugar. Neotame is aspartame plus 3-di-methyl-butyl, which can be found on the EPA's list of most hazardous chemicals.

Unlike aspartame, neotame is not broken down in your body into the amino acid phenylalanine, so it is not toxic to people with phenylketonuria (PKU). But since the chemical structure of neotame is very similar to aspartame, it is logical to assume that many of the other toxicity concerns will still apply.

Stevia

An interesting contrast to the artificial sweeteners discussed thus far is the natural sweetener stevia. Stevia is derived from a South American herb by the name of Stevia rebaudiana Bertoni. Stevia has virtually no calories. Hundreds of tons of stevia extracts have been consumed annually in Japan for almost thirty years with no reported side effects. Since the 1970s, the Japanese have conducted extensive research on stevia, and have found it to be completely safe.[63,64]

Nonetheless, certain countries have refused to certify its use as a sweetener. In the United States, it is banned in food products and beverages and can only be sold as a "nutritional supplement." In Canada, stevia can only be sold as an herb.

Because stevia is natural, it cannot be patented, and so has no chemical corporate interests to generate propaganda in favor of it. The FDA has turned down three requests to allow the use of stevia in foods. Stevia has been the subject of searches, seizures, and embargoes on importation.

Supporters of stevia assert that these actions amount to a restraint of trade designed to benefit the artificial sweetener industry.

Artificial Sweeteners And Weight Gain

A study of artificial sweetener use performed on college students showed no evidence that artificial sweeteners were associated with a decrease in sugar intake. In fact, artificial sweeteners simply perpetuate a craving for sweets, and overall sugar consumption is not reduced—leading to further problems controlling your weight.[65]

Another study showed that drinking both sugar and sugar-free soft drinks increased the likelihood of weight gain by 65 percent, **but it was the diet soda that was associated with "serious weight gain."** This finding was replicated in a study which found that rats fed diet soda ate more high-calorie food than rats fed a drink sweetened with a high-caloric sweetener. According to nutritional expert Leslie Beck, "Your taste buds may be temporarily satisfied by the sweet taste of a diet pop, but your brain isn't fooled, and it still wants to make up for calories later on."[66]

In other words, artificial sweeteners will not even help you lose weight.

"No Calorie Sweetener" Is A Lie

Artificial sweeteners are far sweeter than sugar (and much more expensive), so all powdered artificial sweeteners are mixed with bulking agents like dextrose, sucrose, and maltodextrin to make the sweeteners more palatable, affordable, and easier to handle.

What the unsuspecting public doesn't realize, though, is that these bulking agents are another form of SUGAR.

Dextrose is another term for glucose. This is the same as refined corn sugar. *Maltodextrin* is the scientific term for corn syrup solids composed primarily of fructose and glucose in a starch form.

All artificial sweetener packets are at least 96 percent sugar. And Splenda is even WORSE—99 percent of Splenda® No Calorie Sweetener is sugar.

However, food labeling laws legally allow products to be described as "sugar-free" if the serving size contains less than .5 grams of sugar, and "calorie-free" if the serving size is less than 5 calories. This is why the serving sizes you will see on a bag of Splenda No Calorie Sweetener are tiny: .5 grams (1 tsp.) for the granular and 1 gram for the packets. A 1-gram packet contains 4 calories, but because this is under the 5 calorie rule, it is inaccurately deemed "calorie-free."[67]

More Deception for Diabetics

Research studies have shown that artificial sweeteners, such as sucralose, do not raise blood sugars and therefore are "safe" for diabetics. But there are no research studies to show that the mixture of artificial sweeteners and sugars sold in stores does not raise blood sugars. I suspect these effects were never studied because it was obvious what the results would be: blood sugars would increase.

Dr. Richard Bernstein, a diabetologist with over twenty-three years of experience, in his national bestseller *Dr. Bernstein's Diabetes Solution*, tells all diabetics to avoid powdered artificial sweeteners:

When [artificial sweeteners] are sold in powdered form, under such brand names as Sweet'n Low, Equal, The Sweet One, Sunett, Sugar Twin, Splenda® No Calorie Sweetener and others, these products usually contain a sugar [maltodextrin/dextrose] to increase bulk, and will *rapidly raise blood sugar.*[68]

Conclusion

Artificial sweeteners are perhaps the most extreme example of what has gone wrong with our eating habits. They are beyond processed; they are actually newly created chemicals produced in labs and factories. They serve no purpose other than to satisfy our addiction to something we don't really need to be eating in the first place. They are an attempt to cure our self-created illnesses, but they do nothing but create more disease.

If you are interested in learning more about artificial sweeteners, their history, and the problems they cause, I would suggest my book *Sweet Deception: Why Splenda, NutraSweet, and the FDA May Be Hazardous to Your Health* for further reading (available at Mercola.com).

CHAPTER:

Genetic Engineering
A Most Dangerous Assault on the Future of Food

This chapter was co-written with Jeffrey Smith, one of the world's leading experts in the dangers that genetically modified foods pose to our society.

If you pick up a processed food item at your grocery store, you will most likely be choosing a genetically modified (GM) food. That's because over 70 percent of processed foods contain genetically modified ingredients.[1]

The following 2006 statistics from the U.S. Department of Agriculture's National Agricultural Statistics Service will give you an idea of just how widespread GM crops are in America:

- 89 percent of the soybeans planted in the United States were GM varieties
- 83 percent of the cotton planted was GM
- 61 percent of the corn was GM

Unlike in Europe where processed GM foods must be labeled if any ingredient includes 0.9 percent of genetically modified organisms (GMO) or more, here in the United States, GM foods are not labeled.

In fact, there is a major disconnect between the American public and awareness of GM foods in general. Consider that, according to a 2006 Pew Initiative poll[2]:

- Just 41 percent of Americans say they've heard of GM foods
- Only 26 percent of Americans believe they've eaten GM foods
- In 2006, 60 percent of Americans still believed they had not eaten GM foods

In reality, however, it is not a stretch to say that just about every American has eaten GM foods, whether knowingly or not. Why should you worry if your crackers contain GM corn or your tofu GM soy? Because eating GM foods is, quite literally, like taking part in a giant experiment.

There has only been one study done with humans to show what happens when genetically modified foods are consumed. Animal studies have turned up some disturbing health findings, and these crops are already beginning to infiltrate all of America's soil, meaning that one day, sooner than you think, it may be *impossible* to find foods that haven't been contaminated with GMOs.

What Exactly Is Genetic Engineering, and Why Is It Done?

Back in the mid-1970s, scientists discovered that they could transfer genes from one species to another. This was an unprecedented breakthrough in technology. Of course, through normal sexual reproduction, parents contribute thousands of genes to their offspring. Genetic engineers, however, force a gene (known as a transgene) into the DNA of organisms that could never acquire it naturally. They break the species barrier by creating completely new organisms.

Genetic engineering began so that scientists could implant specific traits into different species, creating crops resistant to pesticides and diseases, foods that can deliver vaccines, and livestock that have more omega-3 fats or other nutritional attributes, among many others. What makes this frightening is that scientists are manipulating animal and plant DNA to create abnormal life forms reminiscent of

Frankenstein. For example, they inserted spider genes into goat DNA so that they could milk the goat for spider web protein to use in bullet-proof vests. Meanwhile, cow genes have turned pigs' skin into cowhide, jellyfish genes have lit up pigs' noses in the dark, and Arctic fish genes gave tomatoes and strawberries tolerance to frost.

Human genes are also being manipulated. Amazingly, pharmaceutical companies have inserted human genes into bacteria, turning them into living factories to produce drugs.

Innovative technological creations, *yes*. Things that are safe to introduce into the human food chain and environment?

Probably not.

Most GM Crops Are Pesticide-Resistant And Highly Contaminated

Adding to the problems surrounding GM crops is that the very thing they've been engineered to do (in many cases this is to thrive even when doused with pesticides) makes them quite toxic. Just five companies comprise the GM seed industry (Monsanto, DuPont, Syngenta, Bayer CropScience, and Dow), and these same five companies also own more than 35 percent of the worldwide seed market[3] as well as 59 percent of the pesticide market[4] (GM seeds from Monsanto, the largest shareholder, accounted for 88 percent of the GM crops planted in 2005).

Out of the four major GM food crops currently being produced (soybeans, corn, canola, and cotton), along with the smaller GM crops (zucchini, crookneck squash, papaya, alfalfa, and tobacco), nearly three-fourths have been engineered to survive applications of a specific herbicide, and nearly one-fifth of them are designed to *produce their own pesticide*. Further, more than one out of ten GM crops do both!

It is no major mystery, then, that when you consume most any GM crop there is a high probability that it has been sprayed with pesticides and, therefore, is highly contaminated. While this is an enormous benefit to food producers, who can spray potentially toxic pesticides freely over their crops without worrying it will harm them, it absolutely fails to factor in the health-damaging effects of the residual pesticides that are consumed by you—nor the incredible damage these pesticides do to the environment.

GM Crops Contain Damaged DNA

Though GM crops may look similar to their natural counterparts, when you look below the surface they are anything but natural. These highly technologic inventions are completely man-made laboratory creations, the likes of which the world has never seen. Even the extremely fragile DNA in these crops is being altered, with completely unknown consequences.

There are two popular methods for creating GM crops, and both interfere with the natural functioning of the plants' DNA. The first method of gene insertion uses a gene gun. Scientists coat millions of particles of tungsten (a metal) or gold with transgenes and then shoot these into millions of plant cells. Only a few cells out of millions incorporate the foreign gene.

The second method uses a bacterium that, under normal conditions, infects a plant by inserting a portion of its own DNA into plant DNA. This causes the plant to grow tumors. Genetic engineers, however, replace the tumor-creating section of the bacterial DNA with one or more genes. The altered bacterium "infects" the plant's DNA with those foreign transgenes instead.

Sound concerning? It is. Unfortunately, you can't simply snap a new gene into place like a Lego and have it function fine. Instead, sections of the plant's DNA near the insertion site are almost always scrambled in some way. Meanwhile, the transgene is commonly shortened, rearranged, or deleted during the insertion process, and plants can end up with multiple copies of the foreign gene, incomplete genes, and/or gene fragments. This can easily set the stage for unexpected consequences.

Further, neither gene insertion method can "aim" the foreign gene into a particular location in the DNA. Because of this, transgenes often end up inside functioning plant genes, changing or destroying them. Yet, scientists rarely conduct experiments to find out where the transgene is and what important natural genes it might have damaged.

Once genes are inserted into the new DNA, scientists typically grow the cell into a fully functioning plant using a method called tissue culture (cloning). Unfortunately, this artificial method of plant reproduction results in *widespread mutations* throughout the plant's genetic structure. In fact, *tissue culture is sometimes used specifically to create mutations* in plant DNA. These mutations can influence the crops' height, resistance to disease, oil content, number of seeds,[5] and other properties that may cause the food to actually become toxic.

The Startling Consequences Of Genetically Mutated Crops

The process of genetic modification easily results in hundreds or thousands of mutations—the changes are vast. Studies have suggested that, conservatively, about 3 percent of the genetic structure of GM plants is different from non-GM plants, yet these differences are not evaluated in the GM food Americans are currently eating.

You and your family have likely eaten a host of GM foods that, by their very nature, contain genetic mistakes and mutations, despite the fact that these mutations carry distinct risks. Among them:

- Causing overproduction of toxins, allergens, carcinogens, or antinutrients
- Reducing the nutritional quality of the crop
- Changing the way that the plant interacts with its environment

And because of our limited understanding of DNA, no one knows what the additional consequences to human health and the environment will be.

The FDA Is NOT Protecting You From These Mistakes

What is extremely important to understand about GM foods is that neither the FDA, nor any other regulatory agency, is monitoring the potential consequences of these creations. The regulatory agencies that approve GM foods operate as if the insertion process has no impact on safety.[6] They do not require extensive evaluation of the mutations, despite the fact that the few studies that have analyzed GM crops *already on the market* reveal significant problems, including:

- Containing scrambled DNA, incomplete genes, or multiple fragments of the inserted gene
- Gene fragments in GM corn that were supposed to be in a different GM crop
- Significant nutritional differences between GM and non-GM crops

Further, GM crops are tested for only a handful of nutrients and known toxins, and therefore, the full extent of the true impact of gene mutations is completely unknown at this time.

Eating Some GM Foods Is Like Eating Pesticides in Every Bite of Your Food

It's not just unpredicted changes in DNA that make GM crops risky. Even the genes that are intentionally added to GM crops may cause harm. Consider the scenario of *Bt* crops.

What are *Bt* crops?

Bt (*Bacillus thuringiensis*) is a soil bacterium that produces a pesticide. Organic farmers sometimes spray solutions containing *Bt* on plants as a natural method of insect control. *Bt* crops, on the other hand, have been altered to contain this pesticide right in their DNA. This way, every cell of these plants produces *Bt*.

Very few studies have assessed the health effects of *Bt* crops. Instead, justification for their approval is largely based on the argument that *Bt* sprays have a history of safe use and that the *Bt*-toxin does not react with mammals. However, research contradicts both arguments.

Bt Crops Cause Harmful Reactions

Bt crops are currently on the market—which means you could be eating them—even though numerous harmful reactions have been reported. In a Monsanto study, rats fed corn engineered to produce *Bt* showed significant changes in their blood, liver, and kidneys, suggesting the presence of disease. Again, this corn is on the market.[7]

When *Bt* pesticide was sprayed in Vancouver to fight gypsy moth infestations, nearly 250 people reported reactions—with mostly allergy or flu-like symptoms. Spraying over the state of Washington resulted in more than 250 health complaints, and workers who apply *Bt* sprays have reported eye, nose, throat, and respiratory irritation.[8] Other reported reactions include eye infections and cornea ulcers,[9] skin irritation, burning, swelling and redness,[10] among many others.

Further, in the United States and Canada, nearly 25 farmers say that certain *Bt* corn varieties caused their pigs to become sterile, to have false pregnancies, or to give birth to bags of water, and a farmer in Germany claims that a variety of *Bt* corn killed 12 of his cows and caused others to fall sick.

The incidences do not end there. In April 2006, more than 70 Indian shepherds reported that 25 percent of the sheep in their flocks died within about one week of continuous grazing on *Bt* cotton plants.[11] Post-mortems conducted on the sheep that ate *Bt* cotton plants showed severe irritation and *black patches in both the intestines and liver* (as well as enlarged bile ducts). The investigating team said the preliminary evidence "strongly suggests that the sheep mortality was due to a toxin . . . most probably *Bt* toxin."

This is not rocket science, folks. The *Bt* toxin is exactly that, a toxic poison that is designed to kill insects. Should it be any surprise that munching on this toxin right in your food would cause serious problems in higher-order animals and humans?

In addition to unpredicted health effects, the *Bt* cotton is having a disastrous impact on the environment. When Monsanto's GM cotton varieties were first introduced in the United States, tens of thousands of acres suffered deformed roots and other problems (Monsanto had to pay out millions in settlements).[12] When *Bt* cotton was tested in Indonesia, widespread pest infestation and drought damage forced withdrawal of the crop despite the fact that Monsanto had been bribing at least 140 individuals for years, trying to gain approval.[13]

In India, inconsistent performance has resulted in more than $80 million in losses in each of two states.[14] And some Indian farmers found that after planting GM cotton, their fields became sterile and could not support subsequent crops.[15] Tragically, thousands of indebted *Bt* cotton farmers from India have committed suicide as a result of the GM crops.

Turning Your Gut Bacteria Into Living Pesticide Factories

Clearly GM crops have had disastrous impacts on animals, but what about on humans? The only human feeding study ever published showed soybeans, that had been genetically modified to make them herbicide-tolerant, spontaneously transferred out of food and *into the DNA of human gut bacteria*.[16] This means that long after we have given up eating GM soy, which is widely available on the market, the bacteria inside our intestines may produce the herbicide-tolerant protein inside of us. If it is allergenic or toxic, it may have long-term effects.

But what is of far more serious concern is that the same study verified that the promoter also transferred to gut bacteria, and the promoter, which is like an on-switch designed to turn on the inserted gene, may turn on genes at random in the bacteria.

GM corn and most GM crops are also inserted with antibiotic-resistant genes. The American Medical Association, the World Health Organization (WHO), and organizations worldwide have expressed concern about the possibility that these might transfer to disease-producing bacteria inside your gut, creating new, antibiotic-resistant super-diseases.

Finally, consider what might happen if the transgene that produces the *Bt*-toxin were to transfer from GM corn into your gut bacteria. It could theoretically transform your intestinal flora into living pesticide factories.

Do You Eat Soy? Then You've Probably Eaten Roundup Ready Soybeans

Roundup Ready soybeans are altered so that Monsanto's popular Roundup herbicide does not harm them. Therefore, farmers are able to apply the pesticide liberally over the GM soybeans so that weeds are killed but the GM soybeans are unaffected. Because of this, much more Roundup herbicide is used on Roundup Ready GM plants than on typical crops.

In fact, by 2004, it was estimated that Roundup Ready acres received 85 percent more herbicide than acres of natural soy. And Roundup herbicide was found to be far more toxic to humans and animals than previously thought.[17]

Soon after GM soy was introduced to the UK, soy allergies skyrocketed by 50 percent.[18] Without follow-up tests, we can't be sure if genetic engineering was the cause, but there are plenty of ways in which genetic manipulation can boost allergies.

- A 1996 study in the *New England Journal of Medicine* confirmed that transgenes could carry allergens from their original species into the GM food.

- Sections of the Roundup Ready protein are identical to those found in shrimp and dust mite allergens.[19]

- In Monsanto's own study, levels of one known allergen, trypsin inhibitor, were as much as seven-fold higher in cooked GM soy and 27 percent higher in raw varieties.

GM Foods Wreak Havoc in Animals

In addition to possible allergic responses, animal studies with GM soy show some extremely serious problems. Mice and rabbits fed Roundup Ready soybeans, for instance, had changes in their liver cells and problems with enzymes in the pancreas, suggesting that GM soy may interfere with digestion.

Even more disturbing results came from a 2005 study conducted by a scientist from the Russian Academy of Sciences. Female rats were fed Roundup Ready soy before conception and continuing through pregnancy and weaning. More than half (55.6 percent) of the offspring died within three weeks compared to 9 percent from female rats fed non-GM soy. Also, many rat pups from GM-fed mothers were significantly smaller, and both mothers and pups were more aggressive. Further, when the GM-fed offspring mated together they were *unable to conceive.*

Bt and Roundup Ready crops are not the only GM foods that have proven to be dangerous to animals. A 1998 study by Rowett Institute scientist Arpad Pusztai found that their GM potatoes caused numerous health problems in laboratory rats.

When the rats were fed the GM potatoes, which had been engineered to produce an insecticide (called GNA lectin), virtually every organ system in the rats was harmed—with most changes found after just 10 days. For instance, compared to rats fed diets with non-GM potatoes (that also contained the natural insecticide):

- Their brains, livers, and testicles were generally smaller, suggesting their normal growth processes had been disrupted due to malabsorption of nutrients or unknown toxins.

- White blood cells responded to a challenge more slowly, indicating immune system damage.

- Organs related to the immune system, including the thymus and the spleen, showed adverse changes.

- The animals had enlarged pancreases and intestines and partial atrophy of the liver.

The GM potatoes also created rapid cell growth in the stomach and intestines of the rats, and the lining of their stomachs and intestines was significantly thicker than controls.[20] Although no tumors were detected, such growth can indicate a precancerous condition. By contrast, rats fed the non-GM potatoes that were spiked with the same lectin were relatively unaffected. Thus, the damage to the rats was not caused by the lectin, but apparently by "the genetic modification process itself."[21]

Quite disturbingly, when Dr. Pusztai went public with these findings and voiced his concerns, he was fired from the job he had held for the last 35 years and silenced with threats of a lawsuit. His 20-member research team was also disbanded and the research stopped. (Unfortunately, this is not unusual. Scientists who discover incriminating evidence or even voice criticism have been threatened, stripped of responsibilities, denied funding or tenure, or fired.)[22]

Hijacked Regulatory Agencies And Rigged Research Puts You At Major Risk With GM Foods

Amazingly, the FDA, which supposedly regulates GM foods, came up with the following statement in their 1992 policy on GM foods:

"The agency is not aware of any information showing that foods derived by these new methods differ from other foods in any meaningful or uniform way."

On the basis of this sentence, the FDA claims that no GM safety studies are necessary. It is now known, however, that the FDA's own scientists had repeatedly warned their superiors that GM foods might create unpredictable, hard-to-detect side effects. They urged political appointees in charge to require long-term safety studies, including human studies, to guard against possible allergies, toxins, new diseases, and nutritional problems.

The scientists' concerns were kept secret from the public until a lawsuit forced the FDA to turn over its internal files, but by then it was too late—GM crops were planted on millions of acres.

The companies that produce GM crops are, of course, not monitoring their safety either. Biotech companies participate in a meaningless voluntary consultation with the FDA, offering only vague research summaries about the crops. Only one crop developer turned in actual feeding study data, for FlavrSavr tomatoes. The GM tomatoes were force-fed to rats (because the rats refused to eat them); several of the rats consequently developed stomach lesions, and **7 out of 40 died within two weeks.**[23]

When 7 out of 40 rats force-fed these tomatoes died, that is a giant clue that there is something desperately wrong with the food. Yet, even though scientists at the FDA agreed the study did not prove the GM tomatoes were safe, political appointees approved the tomato in 1994. (The maker voluntarily decided to put a variety on the market that was not associated with the deaths and lesions, but it has since been taken off the market.)

Those rats are not the only animals that turned away from GM food. Eyewitness reports from all over North America found that when given a choice, cows, pigs, deer, elk, raccoons, geese, squirrels, mice, and rats all avoided GM corn or soy. Do the animals know something that humans don't?

Bovine Growth Hormone And The Dangers In Your Milk

Most industrialized nations have banned genetically engineered bovine growth hormone (rbGH) because of safety concerns. Not so in the United States, where FDA Veterinarian Richard Burroughs said that agency officials "suppressed and manipulated data to cover up their own ignorance and incompetence."[24] He also described how industry researchers would often drop sick cows from studies to make the hormone appear safer. Burroughs had ordered more tests than the industry wanted and was told by superiors he was slowing down the approval. He was fired and his tests were canceled.

In 1998, six Canadian government scientists testified before their Senate that they were being pressured by superiors to approve rbGH even though they believed it was unsafe. They also testified that documents were stolen from a locked file cabinet and that **Monsanto, the drug's maker, offered them a bribe of $1 million to $2 million to approve it.**

Further, a Tampa-based Fox TV station was going to air a series about a potential link between rbGH and cancer. However, just before the series was to air, Fox received threatening letters from

Monsanto's attorney, threatening "dire consequences for Fox News." The show was postponed indefinitely. The reporters who had created the series later testified that they were *offered hush money* to leave the station and never speak about the story again. (They declined.)

Meanwhile, you may have noticed labels on growth-hormone-free milk that state "according to the FDA no significant difference has been shown between milk derived from [rbGH]-treated and non-treated cows." Not only is this statement not true (both Monsanto and FDA scientists have acknowledged an increase in insulin-like growth factor-1, which has been linked to cancer, along with increased pus and antibiotic residues in milk from treated cows), but also it was written by the FDA's former deputy commissioner of policy, Michael Taylor, who, additionally, oversaw the GM food policy. Interestingly, Taylor was previously Monsanto's outside attorney and later became vice president of Monsanto.

GM-Related Health Problems Would Be Hard to Discover

No one monitors human health impacts of GM foods, so if the foods were creating health problems in the U.S. population, it might take decades before we identified the cause. One epidemic in the 1980s provides a chilling example. A new disease was caused by a brand of the food supplement L-tryptophan, which had been *created through genetic modification* and contained tiny traces of contaminants. The disease killed about 100 Americans and caused sickness or disability in about 5,000 to 10,000 others.[25]

The only reason that doctors were able to identify that an epidemic was occurring was because the disease had three simultaneous characteristics: it was rare, acute, and fast-acting. If the GM foods that Americans eat every day created common problems like cancer, heart disease, or obesity, the link to genetic engineering might never be discovered.

The Collapse Of GM Foods

Fortunately, studies show that the more people learn about GM foods, the less they trust them.[26] In Europe, Japan, and other regions, consumers demand that their food supply be GM-free.

In fact, 1 million European Union citizens have recently signed a petition demanding even more GM labeling to protect their foods. While most GM foods are already labeled overseas, food products derived from animals that have been raised on GM feed aren't. So the European consumers are demanding that these products also be labeled—in stark contrast to here in America where GM foods run rampant, but no labels whatsoever are demanded.

But there is a light at the end of the tunnel: if even a small percentage of U.S. shoppers started switching food brands based on GMO content, U.S. manufacturers would respond like their European counterparts.

As such, in collaboration with food manufacturers, distributors, and retailers in the natural products industry, the Institute for Responsible Technology launched an initiative in early 2007 to remove GM ingredients from the entire U.S. natural food sector. Called the Campaign for Healthier Eating in America, this comprehensive program will educate consumers about the health risks of GM foods and promote non-GMO brands through shopping guides. After food manufacturers have had a chance to make the switch, thousands of health food stores will be encouraged to put labels on the shelves next to any remaining hold-out brands that still may contain GMOs.

The Pew opinion poll reported that 29 percent of Americans are already strongly opposed to GM foods and believe they are unsafe. That represents about 87 million people. But even among the 28 million Americans who buy organic food on a regular basis,[27] many do not conscientiously avoid GM ingredients in their non-organic purchases; they usually do not know how.

How To Avoid GM Foods

The Institute for Responsible Technology's initiative will go a long way toward educating consumers about how to avoid GM foods and getting GM foods out of the natural food market altogether. In the meantime, there are several ways to reduce your chances of eating GM foods—you just need to know where to look.

Buying organic is currently the best way to ensure that your food has not been genetically modified. By definition, food that is certified organic must be free from all GM organisms. (Sadly, the spread of GM seeds and pollen is a major concern. So, even organic products may be contaminated with traces of GM elements that have been spread by wind or insects such as bees.)

Reading labels is also important. GM soybeans and corn make up the largest portion of GM food crops, so when looking at a product label, watch out for any soy or corn products, including their derivatives. As mentioned earlier, other GM foods grown in the United States to watch out for include cotton, canola, squash, and papaya.

You Control The Future Of GM Crops

By educating health-conscious shoppers about the dangers of GM food *and* providing clear choices *in the store*, the Institute for Responsible Technology's initiative will give brands without GM ingredients the advantage. This campaign will promote healthier eating in America and may even achieve the tipping point that inspires the whole food industry to get on board. It is up to you, the consumer, to voice your opinions about GM foods contaminating the food supply and make the choice to support non-GM companies. Remember, it will only take a small percentage of Americans to shut down the demand for GM food in America.

To learn more about the Institute for Responsible Technology's initiative, the GM-Free School Campaign, and how to avoid eating GM foods at home and in restaurants, go to www.ResponsibleTechnology.org.

Taking Action

When people realize the extent of the dangers of GM foods, they usually demand that something be done immediately. Many first think of demanding change through the Congress. Although there are U.S. legislators who have introduced bills for labeling and for more extensive testing, these have not yet developed the momentum needed to pass. Check with TheCampaign.org for current news on congressional action.

However, it wasn't legislation that worked in Europe and elsewhere. It was the widespread rejection of GM foods by consumers that forced food manufacturers to remove GM ingredients. Thus, just by taking steps to protect yourself and your family, you are helping to move the market.

In addition, you can help get the word out in your community. One of the most effective methods is to create a GM-Free School Campaign. This program, which is being implemented nationwide, rallies community members around protecting the most vulnerable sector of the population—children. Their young, fast-growing bodies certainly are more sensitive to the potential toxins, allergens, and nutritional problems associated with GM foods. In addition, due to the epidemic of obesity, diabetes, ADHD, and other problems, kids' meals, and especially school meals, are under lots of scrutiny right now. Each school may already have a wellness plan, members of a wellness committee, and plenty of parents actively looking for ways to protect the health of their kids.

The campaign simultaneously alerts a large number of community members, helps educate parents how to buy non-GM brands, is a magnet for local press coverage, and will help to convince food companies that cater to kids and sell to schools to publicly commit to non-GM ingredients.

The Institute for Responsible Technology offers local groups a comprehensive strategy, manual, media kit, their own website and list serves, and materials. Most importantly, the DVD *Hidden Dangers in Kids' Meals* is a tool for "instant activism—just add DVD and stir."

Wherever this 28 minute video is shown, a significant number of audience members want to get involved with the campaign.

In addition to a school focus, there are special roles that people in certain professions can play to advance this cause. Chefs, restaurants, and food companies can switch to non-GM sources, retailers can remove or label GM products or offer in-store Non-GMO Shopping Guides, religious leaders can help to educate their organization and membership, health practitioners can provide patient education materials, and reporters can expose the health risks. The Institute for Responsible Technology offers support for these groups as well.

Although GM foods are among the most dangerous threats we face to our health and to our environment, they are also one of the easiest battles to win. Armed with the facts and clear choices for a healthier diet, we consumers, who are on the top of the food chain, can quickly end this dangerous, uncontrolled experiment.

CHAPTER:

Why Soy is Not a Health Food

In recent years soy has emerged as a "near perfect" food, with supporters claiming it can:

- Provide an ideal source of protein
- Lower cholesterol
- Protect against cancer and heart disease
- Reduce menopause symptoms
- Prevent osteoporosis

However, if you carefully examine the research on soy, you will find that viewing soy as a health food is a distortion of the truth. The reality is that unfermented soy products frequently cause much more harm than good.

So how, then, did soy foods grow from a relatively obscure, seldom-eaten, $800-million industry in 1992 to a mainstream $6.6-billion one expected to grow 5.4 percent annually through 2007[1]—an increase of over 500 percent in a mere 12 years?

The Rise of Soy: From Fringe Product to Disease-Preventive Panacea?

It wasn't too long ago that soy foods were thought of as "hippie" foods or even food for those in impoverished countries. In fact, in 1913 soy was listed in the U.S. Department of Agriculture (USDA) handbook not as a food but as an industrial byproduct.

The "perfect" food that many view soy as today emerged because there are strong corporate influences seeking to profit from the alleged health benefits of soy products like soy milk, powders, soy oil infant formulas, cheese, breakfast bars, cereals, and nuts. At the top of this list is the soy industry itself, which launched an aggressive marketing campaign to convince many health-conscious, trend-setting Americans that soy is the miracle health food that benefits everything from cancer to heart disease to hot flashes—and a slew of other illnesses in between.

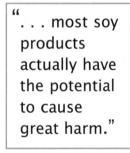

" . . . most soy products actually have the potential to cause great harm."

According to lipid specialist and nutritional pioneer Mary Enig, PhD, the reason there's so much soy in America is because the soy industry started to plant soy to extract the oil, and soy oil became a very large commercial venture that was used to replace many of the healthier tropical oils. Once they had as much oil as they did in the food supply, they had major amounts of surplus soy protein. Since they can't feed this to animals, because anything but small amounts cause health problems in animals, they had to create another market to maximize their profits.

So another market is precisely what the soy industry created. To put it simply, after spending many millions on advertising and intense lobbying with the Food and Drug Administration (FDA) they were highly successful. Their brilliant marketing strategy has convinced nearly three out of four U.S. consumers that soy products are healthy.

So, millions of Americans, many who may have once turned their noses up at the mere thought of soy anything, are now consuming unfermented soy products in record amounts and in newly created, highly processed forms: soy protein shakes, soymilk, soy burgers, soy energy bars, soy ice cream, soy cereal, soy meat—not to mention the soy derivatives present in an overwhelming number of processed foods.

They are convinced that choosing this food will extend their life and prevent many unwanted diseases. Unfortunately, nothing could be further from the truth.

Soy: Too Good to Be True

It's ironic that soy has become so accepted as a health food when, as Dr. Kaayla Daniel, author of the most comprehensive book ever written on this soy deception: *The Whole Soy Story: The Dark Side of America's Favorite Health Food*, states,

> *Thousands of studies link soy to malnutrition, digestive distress, immune-system breakdown, thyroid dysfunction, cognitive decline, reproductive disorders and infertility— even cancer and heart disease.*

Unfortunately, the soy industry has been highly effective in its marketing efforts, and health claims purporting soy's many benefits abound in the media and professional literature. As mentioned, if you listen to all of the hype, soy has been promoted as an ideal source of protein and an excellent way to lower cholesterol, protect against cancer and heart disease, reduce menopause symptoms, and prevent osteoporosis.

This deception was largely facilitated by the soy industry's comprehensive strategy of investing millions in academic research in major universities that supported their contention that soy was a health food. This was done in conjunction with a smear campaign on tropical oils that caused the public and most health care professionals to believe that the saturated fats in tropical oils were evil and should be avoided at all costs.

However, most of the research was fatally flawed, as it failed to separate out the effects of the truly evil fats, trans fats, from the saturated fats. So much of the research that documents adverse health effects from saturated fats was related to the trans fats that were also present in the food.

All the negative PR on saturated fats created a vacuum that was conveniently filled by the domestically grown soy oils. Unfortunately, this monster continued to grow and created ever-expanding markets for soy. Today, the United States cannot meet these growing demands and everyday hundreds of acres of the Amazon rain forest are destroyed so soy can be grown and sold worldwide.

It is tragic enough to destroy the rain forest, as we will destroy plant and animal species that we will never have access to, but the ultimate irony is that the only benefit for this massive destruction is the increase of profits to the edible oil industry. Meanwhile, the health of the world continues to go south because of the negative consequences of consuming unfermented soy.

The Nutrition Committee of the American Heart Association recently examined decades of studies on the health benefits of soy and has found little to no evidence that soy-based foods and supplements significantly lower cholesterol, as is often claimed.

In addition to this inability to demonstrate the beneficial effects of soy on cholesterol levels, the American Heart Association review also found that, contrary to some popular myths:

- Soy isoflavones do not prevent prostate, breast, or uterine cancers as commonly reported.

- Neither soy protein nor soy isoflavones are useful in limiting menopause-related symptoms.

- The jury remains out on any soy-related benefits in treating osteoporosis.

Why Soy Is NOT a Miracle Food

What you frequently don't find mentioned about soy is that it actually contains a number of potentially harmful components and these include:

- **Antinutrients**, which contain inhibitors that deter the enzymes needed for protein digestion. Further, these enzyme inhibitors are not entirely disabled during ordinary cooking. The result may be extensive gastric distress and protein deficiency, which can result in pancreatic impairment and cancer.

- **Hemaglutinins**, which cause red blood cells to clump together and inhibit oxygen uptake and body growth. Soybeans also contain growth-depressant substances (while some of these substances are reduced in processing, they are not completely eliminated).

- **Goitrogens**, which frequently lead to depressed thyroid function.

- **Phytates**, which prevent the absorption of minerals, including calcium, magnesium, iron, and zinc, all of which are co-factors for optimal biochemistry in the body. This is particularly problematic for vegetarians, as eating meat reduces the mineral-blocking effects of these phytates (so it is helpful, if you do eat soy, to also eat meat).

- **Phytoestrogens** (isoflavones) genistein and daidzein, which can mimic and sometimes block the hormone estrogen. These phytoestrogens have been found to have adverse effects on various human tissues, and drinking even two glasses of soy milk daily for one month has enough of the chemical to alter a woman's menstrual cycle. The U.S. Food and Drug Administration (FDA) regulates estrogen-containing products; however, no warnings exist on soy.

- **Aluminum** at high levels. In an effort to remove the antinutrients from soy, soybeans are taken through a series of chemical processes including acid-washing in aluminum tanks. This leaches high levels of aluminum, a toxic metal, into the final soy products.

- **Manganese** at potentially toxic levels. Soy formula has up to 80 times more manganese than human breast milk.

Further, most soybeans are genetically engineered and grown on farms that use toxic pesticides and herbicides like Roundup. In fact, soybeans contain one of the highest levels of pesticide contamination of all foods.

More than 80 percent of soy plants grown in the United States are genetically modified organisms (GMO). One variety alone— Monsanto's Roundup Ready soy—is planted on more than 100 million acres in this country! When you consider that two-thirds of all manufactured food products contain some form of soy, it becomes clear just how many Americans are consuming GMO products, whose long-term effects are completely unknown.

In addition to this, the farmers can use extraordinarily high levels of pesticides because these genetically engineered soy plants contain a gene that makes them resistant to Roundup. Unfortunately, saturating the soy plants with Roundup contaminates not only the soy plants that are eventually placed into the food supply, but also the environment in which the plants are grown, thus further contributing to the environmental toxic burden.

The Potential Health Problems Surrounding Soy

Far from promoting health, most soy products actually have the potential to cause great harm (and this is particularly true when it comes to soy infant formula, which is addressed later in this chapter).

Breast Cancer, Brain Damage, and Infant Abnormalities:

Among the most startling effects is that soy may not prevent breast cancer but may actually increase the risk of breast cancer in women. There is also concerning research that suggests soy can cause brain damage in both men and women, and in infants.

Two senior U.S. government scientists, Dr. Daniel Doerge and Dr. Daniel Sheehan, revealed the above adverse effects and also wrote an internal protest letter, warning of 28 studies revealing toxic effects of soy, mostly focusing on chemicals in soy known as isoflavones, which have effects similar to the female hormone estrogen.

Moreover, they claim that research has shown a clear link between soy and the potential for adverse effects in humans; soy may also lead to health problems in animals including altering sexual development of fetuses and causing thyroid disorders.

The researchers also found that some studies show chemicals in soy may increase the chances of estrogen-dependent breast cancer.

Thyroid Disorders:

Environmental scientist and long-time campaigner against soy-based infant formula, Dr. Mike Fitzpatrick, has warned about the risk of thyroid disease in infants fed soy formula, high soy consumers, and users of isoflavone supplements. Dr. Fitzpatrick cites:

> *There is potential for certain individuals to consume levels of isoflavones in the range that could have goitrogenic effects. Most at risk appear to be infants fed soy formulas, followed by high soy users and those using isoflavone supplements.*

Kidney Stones:

Soybeans and soy-based foods may promote kidney stones in those prone to the painful condition. Researchers from Washington State University measured levels of oxalate in soybeans and soy foods high enough to potentially cause problems for people with a history of kidney stones.

Weakens Your Immune System:

A study published in the Proceedings of the National Academy of Sciences found that genistein, a hormone-like compound found in soy products (including soy-based infant formulas and menopause remedies), may impair immune function.[2] A few reports from the late 1970s and early 1980s also suggested that a soy-based diet impaired infants' immune functions.

Severe, Potentially Fatal Food Allergies:

Soy is a major cause of food allergies, and a Swedish study found that soy, like its botanically related cousin the peanut, could be responsible for severe, potentially fatal, cases of food allergy, particularly in children with asthma, who are also very sensitive to peanuts.

Reduced Fertility:

According to a study involving humans, genistein in soy may impair sperm as they swim toward the egg. Even tiny doses of the compound in the female tract could destroy sperm and decrease fertility. Researchers suggested that avoiding soy around a woman's more fertile days of the month might actually aid conception.

Dangers during Pregnancy and Nursing:

Phytoestrogens in soy produce a variety of mild hormonal actions within the human body, and studies suggest these changes may adversely impact a fetus or nursing infant (including an infant being fed soy infant formula). Among the possible effects to children exposed to too much soy in-utero is an increased risk of breast cancer later in life. Further (although this link needs to be studied further) at least one study has found that soy phytoestrogens increase the risk of birth defects by as much as 500 percent.

Common Soy Myth: Soy and the Asian Diet

It is an undisputed fact that Japanese people live longer than nearly any other culture in the world. You have likely heard the argument that this is primarily related to eating a diet that is high in soy. The truth is that this is just a myth.

First, Japanese people don't eat as much soy as Americans are now eating. One 1998 study showed that a Japanese man typically eats about 8 grams (2 teaspoons) of soy a day, while the average American could easily consume 220 grams (1 cup) of soy from tofu and two glasses of soy milk.

The theory is also flawed because soy in the Asian diet is primarily fermented soy, NOT the highly processed, unfermented, genetically modified and pesticide-contaminated soy that makes up the vast majority of soy consumption in the American diet. There is a huge difference in this respect alone (and I delve into fermented soy and the instances when soy CAN be good for you at the end of this chapter).

The truth is that there are many reasons why Asians typically live longer than Americans; I believe one of the primary reasons has nothing to do with their soy consumption but rather with the ratio of their omega-6: omega-3 fat consumption. The Asian ratio is 3:1, which is very close to the Paleolithic ideal that many experts believe to be about 1:1 for ideal health. Unfortunately, in the United States and in most developed nations, the ratio ranges from 20:1 to 50:1.

As you have seen in Chapter Four on fats, the omega-6:3 ratio is one of the most important elements to optimize in your diet if you are to achieve high-level wellness and avoid disease.

Traditionally, the Japanese have eaten plenty of clean fish, higher quantities of vegetables and much lower quantities of processed foods, which is likely what contributed to their healthy fat ratio. (On a side note, we are already starting to see the longevity of the Japanese decrease, and I suspect that it is due to the contamination of the fish supply with heavy metals like mercury, and chemicals like PCBs.)

Products That Contain Soy: Which Should Be Avoided?

There are many different forms of soy on the market today, soy protein isolate, soybean oil, soy protein concentrate, texturized vegetable protein, and hydrolyzed vegetable protein, to name just a few. As was mentioned earlier, two-thirds of processed foods contain some type of soy product, so you may be eating soy and not even realize it. In fact, soy products are often hidden on labels under ingredient names like bouillon, natural flavor, and textured plant protein.

So among the soy products out there, which are top on my list to avoid?

Soy Infant Formula:

Soy formula is typically given to infants who aren't breastfeeding and have trouble tolerating regular cow-milk-based infant formulas. Nearly 20 percent of U.S. infants are now fed soy formula, which is incredibly concerning as soy infant formula should always be avoided.

The estrogens in soy can irreversibly harm the baby's future sexual development and reproductive health, and it has been estimated that infants who are fed soy formula exclusively receive **five birth control pills worth of estrogen** every day.

In *The Whole Soy Story*, Dr. Daniel explains the dangerous facts about soy that would have any parent seriously concerned—and if the country knew this, the entire population would be up in arms. After all, what could be more reprehensible than harming innocent infants? Consider that:

- Soy *impedes* the sexual maturation of boys.
- Soy *accelerates* the sexual maturation of girls.
- In newborns, the hormonal effects of soy may be irreversible.
- The average daily dose of soy estrogens in soy formula (38mg) is higher than the amounts that cause thyroid problems and endocrine disruption in adults.

And this is not all. Other problems have also been associated with soy infant formula, such as:

- Adverse effects on hormone levels, as it has been associated with reduced testosterone levels
- Impaired thyroid function through isoflavones present in the formula
- Increased risk of behavioral problems

- Exposing infants to up to 2,000 times higher estrogen content than breast milk
- Having potentially high concentrations of aluminum and manganese

Again, I believe soy formula should never be given to infants, as it is nearly guaranteed to cause problems down the road. So if you have a young child or plan to in the future, please avoid soy infant formula at all costs—and spread the word to other parents. Innocent children shouldn't have to suffer so a relatively few soy industry executives can take home fat paychecks.

Soy Milk:

Soy milk has been increasing in popularity in recent years, with sales reaching $1 billion in 2005. Ironically, this now-popular beverage was once nothing more than a waste product of the tofu-making process. Though promoted as healthy, soy milk is a highly processed food that takes several, far from natural, steps to make:

- Soybeans are presoaked in an alkaline solution.
- The resulting paste is cooked in a pressure cooker, which eliminates key nutrients and produces low levels of the toxin lysinoalanine.
- Soybeans may be "deodorized" using a process similar to refining oil.
- Sweeteners (raw cane crystals, barley malt, or brown rice syrup) and flavorings are added to mask any remaining "beaniness" or unpalatable taste.

Aside from being highly processed, it's possible to consume a large amount of soy, which has unknown effects, just by drinking several glasses of soy milk a day. Drinking even two glasses of soy milk daily for one month has enough phytoestrogens to alter a woman's menstrual cycle.

Highly Processed Soy Products:

All non-fermented soy products like tofu, soy milk, and meatless foods made from textured vegetable protein contain anti-nutrients that could potentially harm your health. I recommend avoiding ALL processed soy, including soy protein powders, energy bars, ice cream, cheese, burgers, cereals, and nuts, for optimal health.

How to Avoid Soy in Your Diet

If you would like to eliminate, or at least drastically reduce, unfermented soy in your diet, it will take a little diligence and a bit of homework, but it can be done. The best way is to avoid all processed foods, which will have a multitude of additional benefits as well. Purchase whole foods that you prepare yourself (this means avoiding all pre-packaged, ready-made foods) as this is clearly the best strategy to attain high-level health. The health benefits are clearly worth sacrificing the convenience benefits.

If you do buy processed foods, the Food Allergen Labeling and Consumer Protection Act, which took effect in January 2006, will help. The Act requires food manufacturers to list whether a product contains any of the top eight allergens (soy, milk, eggs, peanuts, tree nuts, fish, shellfish, or wheat), which are responsible for 90 percent of food-related allergic reactions.

If soy is present in a processed food, it must now be listed on the label even if it is present in colors, flavors, or spice blends, and it must be stated in clear language. So if you are looking to avoid soy (or another top allergen) be sure to read food labels diligently.

The Good News Is That Soy Can Be Good for You

We've discussed the many downsides of soy, but it's important to note that soy CAN be healthy—if it is fermented and it is non-GMO (genetically modified). The fermentation process drastically decreases the levels of soy's harmful, anti-nutritive components, and it also aids in liberating otherwise difficult-to-digest nutrients in the soybean, making them more available for absorption.

244

Fermented soy products include:

- Tempeh, a fermented soybean cake with a firm texture and nutty, mushroom-like flavor

- Miso, a fermented soybean paste with a salty, buttery texture (commonly used in miso soup)

- Natto, fermented soybeans with a sticky texture and strong, cheese-like flavor

- Soy sauce or tamari

These products can be found in most health food and in Asian grocery stores. From my review of the literature, consuming fermented, non-GMO soy is the only consistently safe way to achieve the health benefits that are typically touted for consuming soy.

Tofu Is NOT Fermented Soy

You might have noticed that tofu was not included on the fermented soy list. If you are like most people, you probably assumed it was and assumed you would not have the problems

> "Tofu is not natural . . ."

discussed in this chapter. Unfortunately, that is simply not the case.

Tofu is not natural, but rather is a highly processed form of soybean curd—and it has all of the health risks associated with other highly processed soy foods, including potential risks to the brain.

In fact, one study of close to 4,000 elderly Japanese-American men found that those who ate the most tofu during midlife had more than double the risk of later developing Alzheimer's disease.[3] And the 30-year Honolulu-Asia Aging Study found that those who consumed tofu at least twice weekly had more cognitive impairment than those who rarely or never ate the soybean curd.[4]

Soy, such as tofu, may or may not increase the risk of Alzheimer's, as more studies should be done to truly prove this association. But whether or not this is true does not make non-fermented soy any better to consume.

So, stick to the four forms of fermented soy mentioned above (tempeh, miso, natto, and soy sauce or tamari), and pass up the processed soy infant formula, soy milk, soy burgers, soy ice cream, soy cheese, and the myriad of other soy junk foods out there that are so readily disguised as health foods.

CHAPTER:

16

What You Need to Know *Before* Vaccinating

This chapter was co-written with Dr. Isaac Golden, an Australian homeopath who has been researching the effects of vaccinations and homeopathic alternatives for the past 25 years.

Vaccinations are a controversial topic in America, and many individuals have strong opinions either for or against them. In fact, your personal views about vaccines may very well be challenged by reading this chapter, as my own views were challenged over two decades ago.

I first learned of Dr. Robert Mendelsohn, a pioneering University of Illinois pediatrician, in the 1980s. He took a hard line against vaccines,[1] and when I first learned of him 25 years ago, I was quite angry with his work. I truly felt he was promoting criminally inaccurate information and harming the health of millions of children by his strong opposition to vaccines. Interestingly, more than two decades later, I have had those same aspersions cast at me by many physicians.

However, at that time, I was like most skeptics—and my current critics—and believed what I had been told by my conventional medical training (which, of course, was subsidized by the drug companies who profit tremendously from vaccines). I, too, chose to follow the recommendations of my esteemed mentors and was convinced that vaccination was truly one of the greatest inventions of modern medicine.

However, I had made one major mistake: I never bothered to carefully examine the evidence that Dr. Mendelsohn had uncovered to support his position against vaccinations.

During this same time period, the co-author of this chapter, Dr. Golden, was also skeptical of Dr. Mendelsohn's claims about vaccinations. However, he took a different course. Instead of dismissing them, he spent months researching Dr. Mendelsohn's facts to see if his shocking statements about vaccines had any credibility. To his amazement, Dr. Golden discovered that Dr. Mendelsohn's facts were correct and he spent the next 23 years conducting research on alternatives to vaccinations.

Choosing whether or not to vaccinate your child is a very serious decision and one that should not be made lightly. If you currently believe that anyone who opposes vaccination is a quack who should have his or her license removed (as even I believed 25 years ago), then I would encourage you to carefully review the evidence before using "trusted" experts to make the decision for you.

Do You Really Know about Vaccine Safety or Effectiveness?

Billions of dollars have been spent on research into, development of, and promotion of vaccines over the last 50 years. As a result of all this research, or possibly despite it, most national health authorities claim that vaccines are:

1. Responsible for controlling and virtually eliminating most of the dangerous infectious diseases in developed countries

2. Highly effective

3. Extremely safe

4. One of the most cost-effective public health procedures available

5. The only proven method that can prevent infectious diseases

However, if you look closely at the facts, which we'll do later in this chapter, you'll find that each one of these five claims is inaccurate. This does not necessarily mean that vaccination is a dangerous procedure without any benefits at all, but it does raise the important question: **why aren't public health officials completely honest with parents of vaccine-age children?**

Some readers may think this is a strange question, but it reflects the indisputable fact that public health officials are NOT totally honest about the risks and benefits of vaccination. If vaccination was as safe and effective as they claim, then there would be no reason to withhold information, to manipulate research data, and to viciously attack anyone who publicly questions mass vaccination—yet all of these things happen. If authorities only had the best interests of children at heart, there would be no reason for them to dismiss, without objective evaluation, proven options to vaccination. Yet this also happens.

According to a study in the American Journal of Preventive Medicine (AJPM), one-third of parents feel they are not fully informed about the pros and cons of vaccines.[2]

For instance, you may know that vaccines are intended to prevent diseases, but did you know that there are serious risks involved? That children have died from receiving them? That sometimes vaccines aren't effective, and often they contain potentially harmful additives?

If not, you can begin to see where the controversy comes in and why an increasing number of Americans are opting out of vaccinating their children.[3]

Find Me a Physician Who Will Guarantee the Safety of Vaccines

The lack of information surrounding vaccinations makes it essential for parents to inform themselves before vaccinating their children. You, not your doctor, public health officials, or any other medical or government authority, are responsible for this.

In fact, it is sad but true that many parents who conduct their own research become more knowledgeable about vaccination than their family doctor. This, unfortunately, often does not prevent their doctor from criticizing them to the point of being abusive, accusing them of being irresponsible parents because they choose not to vaccinate.

I always tell parents facing such a situation to ask their doctor a simple question:

> *"Will you give me, in writing, your personal guarantee that if you vaccinate my child, the vaccine will be totally effective and totally safe?"*

I have yet to hear of a doctor who would put their personal assets on the line and give such a guarantee. At the same time, I continually hear of doctors who do not hesitate to insist that parents must vaccinate their children and actually become abusive if they are questioned or challenged.

What Is the Best Way to Protect Your Child from Infectious Diseases?

Before delving into the risks and inaccurate claims surrounding vaccines, it is worth asking whether it's necessary to "protect" against infectious diseases in the first place. Some of the diseases against which you vaccinate your child for are, after all, typically harmless and self-limited. Many actually have very mild courses in nearly any healthy child and even have the beneficial effect of building a healthy immune system. For instance, rubella, measles, mumps, and chicken pox can typically be managed easily with good nursing care at home. If given appropriate homoeopathic treatment, the intensity and duration of these diseases can be further lessened.

If your child's immune system is compromised, as it is with many children in third-world countries where there is insufficient nutrition and poor hygiene, then these diseases may be fatal. However, what these children need is good food, clean water, proper sanitation, and a stress-free environment to build up their immune systems—not more vaccines.

It is also true, though, that some infectious diseases that are still present in our communities are potentially very serious. Whooping cough, for instance, is a distressing disease in tiny infants; meningococcal meningitis can be fatal in 48 hours if not properly treated; Hib and pneumococcal disease can both cause great discomfort, and even death from meningitis.

Vaccines against these serious diseases may, then, have a legitimate place in current vaccination programs, but many really do not. And the line between what's a "necessary" vaccine and what's a completely gratuitous vaccine is continually being crossed; as of 2007, the Center for Disease Control and Prevention (CDC) recommends vaccinations for up to 11 different diseases by the time a child is 6 years old![4] Compare that to the early 1950s when vaccinations were given for just four diseases.

And still, there are those who maintain that no vaccine is worth the risks it presents, such as the former director of the National Institute of Health, Dr. James R. Shannon, who said:

"The only safe vaccine is one that is never used."[5]

The bottom line is a simple one: As a parent you hold the ultimate responsibility for the care of your children, and it should be your decision as to what diseases you decide to protect your child against.

This makes a careful consideration of the five vaccine claims made by public health authorities very necessary.

Claim One: Vaccinations Have Virtually Eliminated Infectious Disease

You have likely heard it before:

"Vaccination has been responsible for controlling and virtually eliminating most of the dangerous infectious diseases in developed countries."

There is plenty of evidence that vaccines do have some protective effect. However, this does not necessarily mean that they were responsible for some of the significant reductions in disease levels seen during the 20th century.

In fact, in many cases, disease improvements that have been credited to vaccinations were actually caused by improvements in water quality, sanitation, living conditions and nutrition, which led to an overall increase in public health.

Yet, most health departments will produce data that makes it seem like vaccinations were the savior. How can this be? Take a look at the following two graphs. They include the same set of data—deaths from whooping cough in America from 1923 to 1991—and make it easy to see how statistics can produce false claims about the benefits of vaccination.[6]

Graph 1 shows deaths from the time when mass vaccination against whooping cough began, around 1950. It appears to show that vaccination caused deaths from whooping cough to be virtually eliminated. It certainly has been used by some authors and health officials for this purpose.

However, if you examine the same data from 1900 onward, the data shows unambiguously that **most of the fall in deaths from whooping cough occurred before mass vaccination was introduced!** Vaccination had little, if anything, to do with the reduction, which simply continued at the same rate when vaccination was introduced. Improvements in hygiene, nursing care, and infection control caused the decline in deaths from the disease, not vaccines.

Figure 1

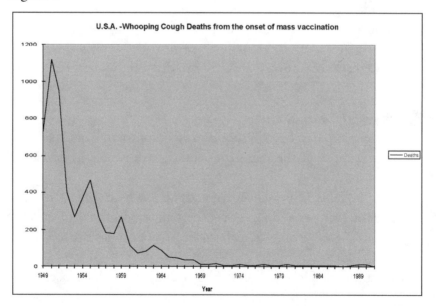

Figure 2

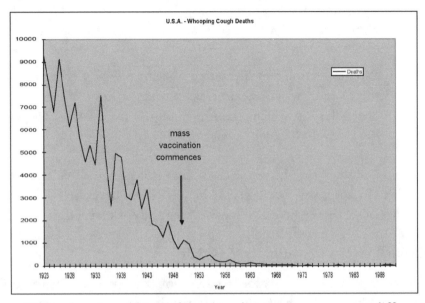

When data is examined for other diseases, even among different countries, most all of them show a similar decreasing trend *before* a vaccine was widely used. Even the widely circulated claims regarding the elimination of polio in the 1950s are greatly exaggerated, as deaths from the epidemics had peaked and were declining before the introduction of an effective vaccine.

Claim Two: Vaccination Is Highly Effective

If you are a parent you were likely encouraged to believe that vaccinating your child would forever protect them from that specific disease. However, even public health sources admit that no vaccine is 100% effective, and most are reported to be between 75% and 99% effective—at best. But these numbers don't even come close to reality, for when you examine real-world outbreaks, as opposed to clinical studies, you will find that protection rates are lower than this. For instance:

- *The Australian Immunization Handbook*[7] states that the pertussis component of the DPT vaccine is 80% effective, but one research study showed an efficacy rate as low as 48.3%.[8]

253

- The measles vaccine is said to be 99% effective after two doses according to *The Australian Immunization Handbook.* However, case reference trials have shown an efficacy as low as 62%.[9]

- Parents are told that the mumps vaccine is 95% effective,[10] yet the efficacy in actual outbreaks can range from **0% to 84%**, depending on which strain of mumps a person was exposed to.

Many studies beyond these also show that, in the real world, vaccine efficacy is well below claimed levels. There have also been bad batches of vaccines where efficacy was zero and/or toxic effects high.

Claim Three: Vaccination Is Very Safe

Parents have every reason to question the potential harm of vaccines. Why? Because a foreign substance is being injected into your child, and many are not aware that this substance can contain potentially toxic chemicals, used to manufacture the vaccine. Routinely used chemicals include mercury and aluminum compounds, both of which are neurotoxins, along with formaldehyde, phenoxyethanol, neomycin, polymyxin, gentamicin, streptomycin, and phenol. Along with these potentially harmful chemicals, some vaccines contain genetic material from animals and humans, including mouse brain serum protein, human albumin, fetal bovine serum, porcine gelatin, and monkey kidney VERO cells.[11]

All of these things are injected into your child during a vaccination, and you deserve to know the risks involved, which can be immediate or may show up much later.

Immediate Severe Reactions to Vaccines

Controlled trials of vaccines show very few immediate deaths or permanent disability. However, these events do occur, as clearly shown by a public health initiative in Japan.

In 1975, following 37 infant deaths linked to vaccination, the Japanese government decided to raise the minimum age for vaccination from 3 months to 24 months in an attempt to reduce the immediate and severe risks associated with giving the DPT vaccine to newborns whose immune systems had not yet matured.

The official Japanese figures, shown in Table 1, have confirmed that immediate severe vaccine damage is significantly reduced by delaying the onset of vaccination.[12] The figures account for episodes for which compensation was paid by the Japanese government and are not the total figures for damage. In fact, it would be safe to assume that they represent only the exposed edge of a large group of damaged children.

Table 1 shows three groups of data, the first being for a period just before the law changed, and the following two for years after the law changed.

Most importantly, the figures show that by delaying the onset of vaccination, the category of Sudden Infant Death Syndrome (SIDS) disappears from the statistics. We expect this result, as SIDS generally only occurs in infants. However, this is clear evidence that vaccination is one cause of SIDS (without being, in any way, the only cause). Other deaths and complications fell dramatically after the minimum age was increased.

Table 1: Comparison of Japanese Vaccine-Related Deaths and Notifications

Year: Period:	1970-1974 61 months	1975-1981 79 months	1981-1984 40 months
Type of vaccine	Whole cell	Whole cell	Acellular
First given	3-5 months	24 months	24 months
Doses (Million)	25.1	19.8	20.4
SIDS	11	0	0
Other deaths	26	3	2
Other reactions	102	39	17

Some people may comment that there are very few deaths and side effects compared to the number of doses of vaccines given. However, for a parent of one of these dead children, statistics are meaningless; only the pain of their suffering matters. We will show below that disease prevention is possible without exposing our children to these potentially tragic consequences.

Vaccination's Long-Term Effects on Overall Health Have Been Understated

You may be surprised to learn that there are practically no long-term studies showing the effect of vaccination on overall health, a glaring omission among the mass of material promoting vaccination.

One exception is research conducted by Dr. M. Odent, later supported and expanded by Dr. Golden's research, which showed negative long-term health effects of vaccination. For instance:

- In 1994, studies by Dr. Odent found that breastfed children who received the pertussis vaccine had a **five times greater chance of developing asthma** in later years than unvaccinated children who were breastfed.

- The vaccinated children had **twice as many ear infections as the unvaccinated children**.

- The vaccinated children were likely to be **hospitalized for longer periods than those who did not receive vaccines.**

Clearly, these findings provide convincing evidence that the long-term risks of vaccination have been understated.[13]

Other articles have indirectly supported Odent's hypothesis regarding a link between asthma and DPT vaccination. Take, for example, a study of over 1,000 children in New Zealand born in 1977. The 23 who were not vaccinated against DPT and polio had no recorded asthma or other allergic illnesses before the age of 10. In the immunized children, 23.1% had asthma, 22.5% had asthma consultations, and 30% had consultations for other allergic illnesses. Similar differences were observed at ages 5 and 16 years.[14]

Dr. Golden's research of asthma, eczema, allergies, and behavioral problems, as well as four types of immunization—homeoprophylaxis

(HP), vaccination, general health measures, and nothing at all—among children aged 4 to 12 years found similar results:

- Vaccinated children were 15.2 times more likely to have asthma than children using homeopathic prophylaxis (HP)

- Vaccinated children were 2.7 times more likely to get asthma than children who used no method of immunization.

- In 19 out of 20 health outcomes measured, vaccinated children were less healthy than children in the other three groups.

So, in terms of overall long-term health, vaccinated children were significantly less healthy in general than all other children.[15] The bottom line? Vaccinations increase your child's risk for developing chronic diseases.

Do Vaccines Cause Specific Diseases like Autism and Alzheimer's?

Diseases such as autism and Alzheimer's have, in fact, been linked to vaccines, but there is a great deal of opposition that keeps the facts from surfacing.

Take, for example, Dr. Andrew Wakefield, whose research in the late 1990s uncovered a link between MMR vaccination and autism.[16] Dr. Wakefield and his team observed that the parents of eight out of twelve children investigated for gastrointestinal symptoms and autism associated the onset of autism with the MMR vaccine.

Even though Dr. Wakefield's research was published in *The Lancet,* one of the most well respected peer-reviewed journals, the medical community was eventually able to have him terminated from his position at the Royal Free Hospital—for no other reason than reporting the truth of his findings about the MMR vaccine.

Dr. Wakefield was not alone in his findings, as other researchers are pointing to the MMR vaccine as being the root cause of the epidemic of neurobehavioral disorders. One researcher in this area, Dr. Vijendra Singh at the University of Michigan, published his findings that a large majority (84%) of autistic children tested had antibodies to myelin basic protein (MBP) in the brain. Moreover, there is a strong correlation between MBP antibodies and antibodies to the MMR vaccine. His findings suggested that exposure to the MMR vaccine may cause the immune systems of children with autism to launch an attack against their own brain cells.[17]

Autism Rates Are Shockingly High Across the U.S. (But NOT Among the Amish!)

The CDC reported that, according to the most recent data available in 2007, a startling one out of every 150 children in the United States has autism.[18] The link between vaccines and this neurodevelopmental disorder is growing every day. The major concern is vaccines that contain thimerosal, a mercury-containing preservative that can harm the brain, particularly in developing children.

Though this toxic additive has been gradually removed from vaccines since 1999, it is still present in some vaccinations, including nearly all flu vaccines (which is why I never get a flu shot and why I advise all people especially children and pregnant women against getting them too).

Thimerosal is incredibly toxic. An Institute of Medicine panel that reviewed data from the CDC's Vaccine Datalink found that children who are given three thimerosal-containing vaccines are **27 times more likely to develop autism** than children who receive thimerosol-free vaccines.

There is also the hard-to-ignore evidence coming from the Amish community, where vaccinations are not typically given. Among the Amish, autism rates are close to nonexistent. When one reporter analyzed a group of Amish children, where, according to rates in the rest of the country, he should have found up to 200 children with autism, he found only three (at least one of which had definitely received a vaccine and developed the disorder shortly thereafter).

In my mind, this provides an irrefutable link to a lifestyle and, most likely, mercury-containing vaccine connection to autism.

According to Dr. Russel Blaylock (RussellBlaylockmd.com), a brilliant neurosurgeon, researcher and consumer advocate:

> *There are research studies on the negative effects of excessive vaccination on a number of organs, especially the brain, as well as clinical evidence of harm. My greatest concern is that hard scientific evidence has shown that excessive vaccination (and children are receiving 34 vaccines before attending school) can significantly alter the developing brain, resulting in a brain that is miswired and, as a result, unable to function on higher levels, as we see in ADHD and autism spectrum disorders.*
>
> *Because the child's brain is undergoing rapid growth and development during the first two years after birth, vaccinations during this time can be especially harmful.*

Alzheimer's Disease: Caused by Vaccinations?

Vaccination has also been linked to Alzheimer's disease. Research conducted at the University of Calgary found that mercury can cause damage consistent with Alzheimer's disease, and one of the main preservatives used in vaccines over decades is, again, the mercury compound[19] thimerosal.

And what is even worse, when an experimental vaccine for Alzheimer's disease was developed, it was found to have life-threatening side effects.[20] So, vaccines may cause Alzheimer's, and a vaccine that was developed to prevent the disease might kill you. Is this evidence of scientific progress?

The list goes on. There has also been, for instance, a long-established relationship between the rubella vaccine and arthritis.[21] Every time new research data is released questioning the safety of vaccines, it is followed by an avalanche of denials, criticism of research methods, and personal attacks on the research scientists involved. The health authorities are not prepared to share the facts with us, so we must uncover them for ourselves.

According to Dr. Blaylock:

> *In the adult, we know that vaccination can greatly aggravate the neurodegenerative diseases, and one study found a 10X increase in Alzheimer's risk in those who receive the flu vaccine 5 years in a row. The public, as well as most physicians, are being kept in the dark concerning this vital research.*

Claim Four: Vaccination Is Cost-Effective

You have also likely heard this claim made by vaccine supporters:

> *"Vaccination is one of the most cost-effective public health procedures available."*

However, what you may not have heard is that conventional medical authorities:

- Have not quantified long-term adverse effects of vaccination
- Stubbornly refuse to objectively evaluate the data available on the homoeopathic option to vaccination
- Have not correctly quantified the effectiveness of vaccination

Therefore, it is impossible to make "scientific" claims about the cost-effectiveness of vaccination. Yet grand claims are made and are picked up by politicians who allocate massive public funding to subsidize vaccination.

So it is important to ask, "Why do health authorities relentlessly push vaccination, and if health authorities have nothing to hide, why do they feel the need to selectively quote and manipulate data?"

Follow the Money Trail—Vaccinations Are a $3-Billion Industry

That's right, $3 billion. With so much money at stake, why *wouldn't* the vaccine manufacturers and pharmaceutical companies lobby for compulsory vaccinations for all children? These same pharmaceutical companies use their money and power to influence and control our government and medical schools, indoctrinating physicians and politicians that vaccines are essential to preventive medicine and health.

According to Dr. Blaylock:

> *There is abundant evidence from a number of sources showing that the present vaccine program is abundantly dangerous for both children and adults. Practicing physicians, medical board members making vaccine recommendations, and lawmakers enforcing their recommendations have no clue as to the deleterious effects of the present vaccine program on brain development and neurodegenerative diseases.*
>
> *They are being misled by vaccine manufacturers and physicians supported financially by these manufacturers into believing these vaccines are perfectly safe.*

Vaccines are also the bread and butter of the pediatrician's practice. Interestingly, pediatricians earn the lowest income of any specialty, and without vaccines, many would suffer financial hardship. In fact, if too many parents stopped vaccinating their kids, many pediatricians would have to shut down because they could not afford to stay open.

Beyond the money, some believe there is evidence to support the fact that our government has an agenda to weaken the population, as there is a never-ending pattern of failure to protect the public from toxins in our food and drug supply. According to Dr. Blaylock:

> *Despite the great deal of evidence that shows that vaccinations are dangerous, our government run schools make vaccinations mandatory for attendance. Our government also has done nothing to stop the use of concentrated excitotoxins in foods and drinks. It is agreed among neuroscientists that excitotoxins damage neuronal pathways and connections and can even kill neurons themselves, thereby aggravating a great number of excitotoxin-related disorders- such as Alzheimer's dementia, Parkinson's disease, strokes,*

brain trauma, multiple sclerosis, autism, ADHD and mercury toxicity.

*One can only conclude that either they are totally irresponsible and ignorant of the work of their own scientists or they are **purposefully dumbing down the population.** By doing so, they would create a population that was so apathetic they would be willing to accept any government agenda, no matter how nefarious.*

There is simply too much at stake to allow the public to know the full truth about vaccinations.

Claim Five: Vaccination Is the Only Way to Prevent Infectious Disease

It is probable that many people choose to vaccinate themselves and their children because they believe the claim that "vaccination is the only proven method that can prevent infectious diseases."

However, what you as a parent need to understand is that you can help to protect your children against all types of infectious diseases by providing them with healthy food to eat. Also important is eliminating processed foods and sugar as much as practically possible, as these foods typically lead to immune system impairment that will subsequently increase the risk for developing these infections.

Research published over 50 years ago beautifully illustrates this fact. When scientists attempted to infect healthy rabbits with polio, they were unsuccessful until they started to feed the rabbits sugar.[22]

Providing children with a peaceful and loving home environment will also enhance general wellbeing and support good nutrition.

Homeopathic Immunization: A Safe and Tested Alternative to Vaccination

If your aim is to maximize your child's immune defenses against a particular infectious disease, evidence shows that this can be done by combining good nutrition with homeopathic immunization (or *homeoprophylaxis* (HP), which uses disease-specific remedies that are non-toxic but provide a level of protection comparable to vaccines.

HP was first used in the late 1790s and has a 200-year history of substantial effectiveness in epidemic situations around the world. Commencing in 1985, Dr. Golden has conducted the world's largest trial of the long-term use of HP against common childhood diseases. His research has demonstrated a level of effectiveness of around 90%, with positive long-term health effects.

There is a considerable body of research evidence supporting these findings, and if you are interested in learning more, it's available either via his Web site, www.homstudy.net, or in his major publication *Vaccination & Homoeoprophylaxis? A Review of Risks and Alternatives, 6th edition.* Dr. Golden's 15 years of research show that a five-year HP program has been effective for disease prevention for the following six potentially serious diseases:

- Whooping cough
- Polio
- Tetanus
- Meningococcal disease
- Pneumococcal disease
- Haemophilis influenzae type B (Hib)

As a Parent, it's Your Right to Make an Informed Choice

Whether or not parents choose to use the HP program in conjunction with better nutrition, every parent who decides not to vaccinate their children should become fully informed of their rights to obtain religious or philosophical exemptions. (These rights have been thoroughly covered on my Web[23] site and in Appendix A.)

As I said at the beginning of this chapter, the decision concerning vaccination is one of the most difficult that any parent has to make. Unfortunately, most parents are unable to make an informed choice because they are not given all the facts. It is important that you have an opportunity to see evidence regarding the safety and effectiveness of vaccines and know that you have the legal right to refuse them, as well as see the evidence supporting the homoeopathic alternative. You now have the information you need to make a thoughtful and informed decision for the future health of your child.

Note: People who are interested in obtaining Dr. Golden's long-term homeopathic immunization program may contact him on admin@homstudy.net, and he will forward your details to the appropriate practitioner. The five-year program costs around $100.

CHAPTER:

Personal Care Products
The New Chemical Warfare

Sharon gets her hair colored every few months with a dazzling red-brown hue. She can always detect the smell of the hair color and notices that her scalp tingles a bit while having it done but knows the sensation will pass. To preserve her color she uses a color-enhancing shampoo every other day and uses extra-hold hair spray to reduce fly-away hair and give it some extra shine.

She buys her make-up and most of her skin-care products from department stores but thinks it's a little strange that she can't find a single ingredient on some of the packaging. The label on her package promises to regenerate her skin cells, and even though her lipstick tastes funny, she loves to reapply it throughout the day.

Sharon uses tartar control fluoride toothpaste and rinses her mouth out with a cool mint mouthwash. She uses a scented shower gel, wears a sunscreen from the drugstore under her moisturizer, and loves to slather on her favorite body lotion every day after taking a shower because it smells like kiwi. She gives herself a few sprays of "Obsession" before getting dressed & uses deodorant that she purchased from the drug store because that's all that works for her. She loves manicures & pedicures and uses an assortment of nail polish regularly.

She disinfects her bathroom frequently with bleach, dusts weekly with furniture polish, and cleans with a bright purple spray cleaner that has lavender listed as a primary ingredient; she can't pronounce the next five ingredients on the bottle. Sharon has the perfect cocktail of carcinogenic (cancer-causing), neurotoxic (brain toxins) and teratogenic (toxic to reproductive organs) products that she invites into her bloodstream on a daily basis.[1]

Sharon is also pretty sedentary and can't remember the last time she broke a sweat while exercising. Her water intake is minimal and she drinks it when she remembers to. Sharon does most of her shopping at Jewel and does not prioritize organic food. Sharon suffers from chronic fatigue, dermatitis, constipation, mental fog, and has difficulty breathing at times. Her doctor recently found a mass in her right breast and would like her to come in for a mammogram.

Toxins are filtered in your liver but are stored in fat tissue. Sharon is exposed to a plethora of toxins and does not engage in any type of detoxification such as sweating or adequate elimination and spends very little time outdoors. Sharon also has the added assault of ingesting pesticide residues, food additives, and excess estrogens from animal drugs in her beef and chicken in addition to her unsafe personal care products.[2]

This is just one scenario among many individuals who are unaware of their own toxic overload.

It may be hard to conceive the possibility that most personal care products designed to intoxicate your senses with fragrant, neatly packaged, and appealing marketing slogans may actually cause cancer, promote brain toxicities and damage our reproductive organs.[3,4]

As illustrated in Sharon's daily encounter with chemical warfare, we regularly mirror this scenario as a result of the blind trust we give to the very agencies designed to protect us.[5] In order to protect and improve our existing health and environment, it is critical for us to be selective in all areas of personal care.[6]

You do not need to understand the language of a chemist to become a discerning consumer when shopping for personal-care products. Let the following information be a guide to you and your family when making personal-care selections, and please remember that anything you put on your skin can be absorbed into your bloodstream, so if what you are putting on your skin contains toxic ingredients, you will be insidiously poisoning yourself.[7]

Cleaners:

▼ *Beware of:* chlorine, chloroform, diethanolamine (DEA), triethanolamine (TEA), and aerosols due to the tiny particles that are easily inhaled.[8]

Keep in mind that indoor air pollution can far exceed the number of toxicities you are exposed to when compared to outdoor pollution, so take the necessary precautions to keep your indoor air as safe as possible especially in the winter and in poorly ventilated areas.[9]

Safe alternatives: Consider buying non-toxic cleaners such as Ecover, Earthrite and Bon Ami. Or to make your own non-toxic cleaner-for cleaning bath, sink, tile, tabletops etc: 2 tsp borax powder, 2 T distilled white vinegar or lemon juice, 3 drops eucalyptus or lavender oil, 2 cups hot water. Optional: add in 1/4 cup of Dr. Bronner's liquid castile soap and place in a spray bottle.

Another way to improve the air quality in your home: adorn your living space with plants that clean the air such as Areca or Lady Palms, Boston ferns, and Rubber plants.[10]

Laundry Detergent:

▼ *Beware of:* formaldehyde and ethoxylated alcohols.[11]

Safe alternatives: Dr. Bronner's Pure Castile soap, EarthRite, and Ecover.

Shampoos and Conditioners:

▼ *Beware of:* artificial fragrance, ingredients such as DMDM hydantoin, and polyethylene glycol (when combined produce formaldehyde as a by-product), sodium lauryl or laureth sulfate and artificial colors such as FD&C Blue 1 or FD&C Red 40.[12]

Safe alternatives: Aubrey Organics, Weleda, or Logona. Add beautiful shine to hair by adding a few drops of peppermint essential oil to your conditioner and work your scalp for two minutes. Rinse with tepid water. Use 1/2 cup raw apple cider vinegar as a final rinse at least once per week to help remove build-up.

Deodorant:

Beware of: aluminum chloride, propylene glycol, and methyl and propyl paraben.[13]

Safe alternatives: LeCrystal roll-on, Nature DeFrance French clay, or Weleda sage deodorant. Two parts of pure water to one part apple cider vinegar along with a few drops of tea tree oil and/or lavender oil can be kept in a spray bottle as a natural deodorant.

Liquid and Bar Soap:

Beware of: parabens, propylene glycol, sodium lauryl and laureth sulfate, artificial fragrance, and fatty alcohols.[14]

Safe alternatives: Dr. Bronners castile bar and liquid soap, Kiss My Face olive oil bar soap, Aubrey organics, Aura Cacia, and Chica Bella.

Toothpaste and Mouthwash:

Beware of: sodium lauryl or laureth sulfate, alcohol, polysorbate 80, and artificial colors such as FD&C Blue 1 or FD&C yellow 5.[15,16]

Safe alternatives: Peelu toothpaste, Ecodent toothpowder, Weleda pink toothpaste, and Xylifresh. Make a paste with 1/2 teaspoon of baking soda and a dash of celtic salt for an effective and non-toxic toothpaste alternative.

Safe mouthwash alternatives: Logona herbal mouthwash concentrate, Weleda, or Xylifresh. For a natural mouthwash, combine two drops of tea tree oil or peppermint essential oil along with 1/2 cup of pure water. Rinse for 60 seconds.

Make-up:

☠ *Beware of:* Aluminum, Talc, propylene glycol, D&C Red 33, FD&C Yellow 5, DEA, TEA, quaternium 15 and 2-bromo-2-nitropropane-1,3 diol (can produce formaldehyde when broken down), and isopropyl myristate which can produce carcinogenic nitrosamines as a result of being combined with NDELA (n-nitrosodiethanolamine).[17,18]

Safe alternatives: Dr Hauschka (pigments from flower petals are used for color), Ecco Bella, Aubrey Organics, Gabriel, Larenim mineral make-up, and Hemp Organics.

Hair-color:

☠ *Beware of:* phenylenediamine, Acid Orange 87, Solvent Brown 44, Acid Blue 168, Acid Violet 73. It is important to remember that black, red, and brown hair dyes are highly carcinogenic.[19]

Safe alternatives: Henna, decoctions made with henna, chamomile, walnut, and black walnut as color enhancers, Ecocolor, and Naturetint (contain phenylenediamine but a very small percentage when compared to conventional hair color).

Skin-Care:

☠ *Beware of:* propylene glycol, parabens, sodium lauryl or laureth sulfate, quaternium 15, imidazolidinyl urea, DMDM hydantoin (can release formaldehyde), and artificial colors.[20]

Safe and effective alternatives: MyChelle, Arcona, Dr. Alkaitis, Trilogy, and Aubrey Organics. Combine equal parts of strongly brewed green tea and raw milk; apply with a cotton ball to add luster and tone to skin. Combine 1 tsp fresh ginger juice, 2 tbsp watercress juice, 1/2 tsp lime or lemon, and apply with cotton to promote skin circulation, maintain clear skin, and speed up the healing process. For dry skin, make a cleanser with raw cream combined with freshly squeezed orange juice, and work the mixture into your skin for 60 seconds; then, rinse with tepid water. Using acupressure facial points and doing daily facial exercises also work wonders for improving and maintaining the tone of your skin.[21]

CHAPTER:

Seven Common Health Myths

There is an overwhelming amount of health information circulated by the media, and it can be difficult to sort through what is credible and what is not. What's more, some of the information that has been accepted as truth by many experts, health care practitioners, and Americans are actually myths.

Your health really depends on your own ability to sort through all of the information and pick out what is reliable. Unfortunately, you often cannot rely on the "popular" opinions to give you the best results. Here are six common health myths that are wrongly accepted as truths by many.

Myth #1: If You Get Sick, Your Doctor Can Solve Your Problem with Drugs and Surgery

Drugs, surgery, and hospitals are rarely the answer to chronic health problems. Care, not treatment, is the answer. As you have been reading about in this book so far, the key to facilitating the natural healing capacity that all of us have is to improve your lifestyle, diet, and exercise.

Nonetheless, many people immediately assume that a drug or medical procedure is the necessary "cure" for their illness. This prevailing myth in our society has led to countless unnecessary medical procedures (and associated side effects).

According to a definitive review compiled by careful analysis of medical peer-reviewed journals and government health statistics, Gary Null, PhD and colleagues, the annual number of:

- Unnecessary medical and surgical procedures performed: 7.5 million.

- Unnecessary hospitalizations: 8.9 million.

- Iatrogenic [induced inadvertently by a physician or surgeon or by medical treatment or diagnostic procedures] deaths: 783,936. This is the equivalent of five 747 jumbo jets crashing every day for a year. If this were the case, would you ever fly?

Further, a 2006 study in the *Journal of the American Medical Association* found that more than 700,000 people, especially those 65 and older, visit U.S. emergency rooms each year as a result of adverse drug reactions.[1] (This is actually a *very low estimate* because a large percentage of drug reactions are misdiagnosed.)

Bear in mind that this study does not only apply to prescription drugs, but also to over-the-counter drugs, vaccines, vitamins, dietary supplements, and herbal products.

The bottom line is that only by addressing the underlying causes of illness can you achieve the answer to your health care challenges; anything else is nothing more than a potentially dangerous symptomatic band-aid. Drugs and surgery, far from solving the real problem, serve as a symptom reliever that is designed to increase corporate profits at the expense of your long-term health.

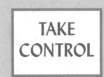
TAKE CONTROL

No More Acne After Thirty Years Of Failed Drug Treatment

After fighting with acne since the age of 13, taking countless antibiotic prescriptions including

4 or 5 series of Accutane, I read Dr. Mercola's Take Control of Your Health Program. At this point, I was ready to try anything and began to cut out processed grain products and sweets. I am 45 years old now and finally have clear skin for the first time in 32 years!

—*Margaret Scrivens, Calgary, Canada* ❧

Myth #2: Over-The-Counter Medications Are Completely Safe

Each year, Americans purchase about *5 billion* over-the-counter (OTC) drugs in the hopes of treating routine medical problems. Many believe OTC drugs do not pose the same risks as prescription drugs and are completely safe to use, as they are so readily available.

Unfortunately, the ease with which OTC drugs can be obtained presents a false sense of security. As with all drugs, OTC drugs are merely covering up symptoms and are not addressing the underlying cause of disease.

Furthermore, even though they're available without a prescription, OTC drugs are still drugs and frequently are simply lowered doses of drugs previously only available by prescription. Over-the-counter drugs have the potential to cause serious side effects and can even result in death if taken incorrectly.

Some 56,000 people end up in the emergency room each year from liver damage due to acetaminophen, the active ingredient in Tylenol. As with prescription drugs, OTC drugs can interact with foods, other medications, and existing medical conditions and cause additional complications.

It's also possible to easily overdose on OTC medications without even knowing you have done so. For instance, according to government estimates, about 100 people die each year after unintentionally taking too much acetaminophen (an overdose of the drug, which includes Tylenol, can poison the liver). In early 2007, the government required new warning labels on OTC cough preparations as three infants were killed by consuming over 14 times the therapeutic level of pseudoephedrine. Many hundreds of others were not killed but had to be treated in emergency rooms.

One of the biggest problems is that many OTC medicines sold for different uses have the same active ingredient. So, someone who takes a cold remedy along with a headache remedy or prescription pain reliever may be inadvertently receiving three or four times the safe level of certain ingredients. Thus, you should check labels to make certain you are not taking multiple drugs with the same active ingredient at the same time.

Along with acetaminophen, another group of OTC drugs to watch out for are painkillers called NSAIDs (nonsteroidal anti-inflammatory drugs). Some of the more common ones include aspirin, ibuprofen, naproxen, and ketoprofen. Overdosing on these widely available drugs can cause stomach bleeding and kidney problems.

While OTC drug labels include some of the potentially harmful interactions on the label, you cannot rely on labels to cover every harmful interaction. Certain foods, drugs, herbs, vitamins, and your own existing medical conditions could potentially create a harmful reaction.

A useful way to learn about these potential interactions would be to talk to a doctor or pharmacist, but since many OTC drugs are sold in grocery stores, convenient stores, and even gas stations, there isn't always a knowledgeable person available to answer your questions.

There are many interactions that can occur and many that are unexpected. For instance, if you have high blood pressure, you could have an adverse reaction if you take a nasal decongestant.

Most consumers also don't realize that vitamins and herbs can interact with medications just as medications can interact with each other. Interactions could cause unexpected side effects, could alter the effectiveness of the drug or vitamin making them more or less powerful, or could even worsen the condition being treated.

Finally, many OTC medications contain additives that may surprise you, such as artificial dyes, caffeine, and artificial sweeteners like aspartame or sucralose. You will want to be sure to read the inactive ingredients on the label along with the active ingredient section to be sure you are aware of exactly what you are consuming.

Myth #3: Fluoride Is Beneficial in Your Toothpaste and Drinking Water

Imagine a drug prescribed to the entire U.S. population with no consent and no way to track dosage or individual reactions and with no concern for some people's increased vulnerability to the drug. It sounds crazy, but that is exactly what is happening in the United States with water fluoridation.

Fluoride has been added to the U.S. water supply for over 50 years in order to "prevent dental decay." Not only is this practice unsafe, but to add insult to injury, it is also ineffective. Data compiled by the World Health Organization shows absolutely no difference in tooth decay in countries that use fluoridated water compared with countries that don't use fluoridated water.[2]

Furthermore, several additional studies have found that tooth decay rates do not increase when water fluoridation is stopped and, in some cases, the rates even decrease.

The largest U.S. survey ever done on this subject, conducted from 1986 to 1987, found that fluoridated water made no difference in tooth decay when measured in terms of DMFT (Decayed, Missing, and Filled Teeth), and made a statistically insignificant difference (on about 0.5 percent of 128 tooth surfaces) when measured as DMFS (Decayed, Missing, and Filled Teeth Surfaces).

When water fluoridation first began, it was believed that fluoride had to be ingested for it to be effective. However, this has since changed, and the dental community now nearly uniformly believes that fluoride's benefits result from topical application, not when it is swallowed.

Despite fluoride's apparent ineffectiveness, it continues to be used in the United States, but not without consequences. The fluoride that you ingest from the water supply and from a number of other sources such as toothpaste, mouthwashes, processed food, some vitamin tablets, and beverages like fruit juice, soda, and tea is associated with a number of negative health effects. Consider that fluoride:

- Accumulates in your bones, making them brittle and more easily fractured.

- Accumulates in your pineal gland, which may inhibit the production of the hormone melatonin, which helps regulate the onset of puberty.

- Damages tooth enamel (known as dental fluorosis) and may lower fertility rates.

- Has been found to increase the uptake of heavy metals such as aluminum and lead into the brain and bloodstream.

- Depresses your immune system by inhibiting antibodies from forming in the blood.

- Confuses your immune system, causing it to attack the body's tissues. This can increase the growth rate of tumors in people prone to cancer.

Noting these and other health risks and the obvious ethical issue of medicating an entire population without their consent, many European countries have banned water fluoridation.

To put it simply, fluoride is not the beneficial additive that is purported to be. This is why, if you look on a tube of fluoride toothpaste, you will see a warning label. There is enough fluoride in a typical tube of toothpaste to kill two small children if they consumed the entire tube all at once. Clearly not something you want to be ingesting regularly!

Myth #4: Cell Phones Are Safe

In 2006, close to 1 billion NEW cell phones were sold. Nearly every adult in a modern country seems to own one, so the issue of whether or not they contribute to brain damage, cancer, or other health problems is quite significant, as the majority of the population could be harmed.

Media headlines seem to jump back and forth between reporting on the dangers of cell phones and then reporting on their safety, but it is my belief that cell phones are capable of causing harm.

Cell phones can wreak havoc on your brain by exposing it to harmful radiation and electromagnetic fields. Though studies are often conflicting, cell phones have been associated with:

- Exciting the brain cortex nearest to the phone, which could potentially cause seizures.
- Increasing the risk of brain cancer and brain tumors.
- Lowering sperm count in men.

Very few readers of this book are old enough to remember the *Journal of the American Medical Association* ads that showed physicians smoking and describing all the health benefits of smoking in the 1920s. Nearly 100 years later, after science has had time to document the destructive effects of tobacco, these ads look absolutely ridiculous. I suspect many "experts" voicing denial of cell phone radiation damage are similarly in denial and don't want to face the reality that they may need to reduce their cell phone radiation exposure.

So, it is my projection that not too far down the road, many of the expert articles you have read defending how safe cell phone use is will be viewed as equally ridiculous as the 1920 JAMA cigarette ads are viewed today.

The first step in protecting yourself from the negative health effects of cell phone use is to put some distance between you and the phone. The best is to use a cell phone with a speakerphone and not hold the phone or put it on your body. If this is inconvenient, then a headset can be used.

Any headset is better than no headset, so if you have one, use it. I have carefully examined this issue, though, and found that many experts are concerned that the cell phone radiation can actually travel down the headset wire to your head. If you use a cell phone at all, I would highly recommend using one that has an air tube to prevent the radiation from traveling to your brain.

Personally, this is the type I use almost all the time. If I don't have it with me, I use my speakerphone, but I refuse to place a cell phone against my head. I also attach a ferrite magnetic bead that surrounds the cell phone wire and further reduces radiation exposure.

Myth #5: Microwave Ovens Are Safe

Microwave ovens may be convenient (an estimated 90 percent of U.S. homes have them), but there's a reason why I haven't had a microwave in my kitchen for over 15 years and—much to the disappointment of my employees—pulled it out of the office many years ago.

This is something that you probably already intrinsically suspect but don't want to acknowledge due to the convenience factor.

What is wrong with microwaves? Microwaves heat your food by causing it to resonate at very high frequencies. While this can effectively heat your food, it also can cause changes in the chemical structure of the food that can, in turn, lead to health problems.

Heating food can cause problems in and of itself because many micronutrients are heat sensitive and will be destroyed in the heating process, but when you heat food with microwaves, you have the additional problem of the creation of potentially negative energy frequencies that further devitalize your food, and possibly your body, once you consume them.

This is one of the possible explanations for the following observations:

- A study published in the November 2003 issue of *The Journal of the Science of Food and Agriculture* found that broccoli "zapped" in the microwave with a little water lost up to 97 percent of the beneficial antioxidant chemicals it contains.[3] By comparison, steamed broccoli lost 11 percent or fewer of its antioxidants.

- The temperature of microwaved food can become extremely hot, at temperatures high enough to cause burns or steam buildup that could explode—this is especially risky with baby bottles. Plus, microwaving can break down the essential disease-fighting ability of breast milk to protect your baby.

- A 1991 lawsuit involved a woman who had hip surgery and died because the blood used in her blood transfusion was warmed in a microwave. Blood is routinely warmed before transfusions, but not by microwave. The microwaved blood caused her death.

- Additionally, when microwaving, carcinogenic toxins could be leached from your plastic and paper plates or covers and mix with your food.

Myth #6: The FDA Is Your Protector

Please be especially careful about this major myth. It is important for you to quickly realize that as currently configured, the FDA is simply UNABLE to adequately protect you because of a massive conflict of interests. The FDA is more interested in protecting the interests of its client: the drug industry.

Like it or not, that is the way the FDA is currently structured, and the sooner you understand that, the safer you and your family will be.

Within the Center for Drug Evaluation and Research, about 80 percent of the resources are geared toward the approval of drugs and 20 percent is for everything else. Drug safety is a measly 5 percent. This speaks loads about the FDA's priorities. The FDA is NOT about protecting you and your family; it is about approving drugs as quickly as possible so the drug companies can reap their profits.

To add insult to injury, Congress enacted the Prescription Drug User Fee Act (PDUFA) 1992, by which drug companies actually pay money to the FDA so they will review and approve their drug. This creates a massive conflict of interest and fox-guarding-the-henhouse phenomena.

PDUFA was enacted 13 years ago and passed by Congress as a way of providing the FDA with more funds. This way, it could hire more physicians and other scientists to review drug applications so drugs could be approved more quickly.

You see, every day that a drug is held up from being marketed, drug companies lose about $1 million to $2 million. Yes, you read it correctly, $1-2 MILLION for every DAY the drug is held up from being approved.

So, the obvious incentive is to approve drugs as quickly as possible and not stand in the way of profit-making.

Additionally, if you think for a moment that the superficial warnings the FDA mandates for certain drug labels are going to have any influence on the way they are prescribed, think again. This is merely a ploy by the FDA to appease the public and appear that they are doing their job. These warnings have been proven time and time again to make absolutely no difference in prescribing rates.

The FDA administration is a massive conflict of interest, with top officials shuttling back and forth between jobs in government and jobs in the industry they're supposed to be regulating. So, please wake up and face the reality (if you haven't already done so) that it's up to you to assume total responsibility for your health and the health of your children. The government is simply not going to do it for you.

Myth #7: There Is No Reason to Worry about Food Additives in Processed Foods Because They Are Present in Such Small Amounts

Food additives, which include everything from artificial colors, artificial sweeteners, preservatives, and flavor enhancers like monosodium glutamate (MSG), are added to just about every processed food (i.e. anything that comes in a bag, box, can, or wrapper). They're used to make foods taste better, extend shelf life, improve texture, add color . . . you name it, there's probably a food additive that does it. But far from being the inert substances that food manufacturers claim they are, food additives are ripe with unhealthy side effects.

The cumulative effects of consuming chemical food additives are largely unknown, but already problems are surfacing:

- A common flavoring called methyleugenol, which is found in many foods and spices, has been connected to causing cancer of the liver, stomach, and kidney in mice and rats.[4] Some of the common foods this flavoring can be found in include candy, cookies, bubblegum, pumpkin pie, puddings, ice cream, apple butter, chutney, anise biscotti, French toast, ketchup, nutmeg, and gingerbread.

- A common blue food dye may have caused the deaths of two patients after it was used to color the liquid food pumped into their stomachs according to a report in the New England Journal of Medicine.[5] The patients had been given food with FD&C blue dye No. 1, after which their skin and blood turned a bluish-green. Several hours later, the patients, a 12-month-old with Down's Syndrome and a 54-year-old with kidney failure, were dead.

- Sodium nitrite, a preservative commonly used in processed meats such as beef jerky and luncheon meat, has been found to break down into cancer-causing chemicals during digestion.

One of the worst offenders when it comes to food additives is the flavor enhancer monosodium glutamate (MSG), which is added to countless processed foods. MSG is a toxic substance, and most people probably would think twice about eating it if they knew it actually causes many of their brain cells to die.

MSG, like L-cysteine and aspartame, are excitotoxins, chemical transmitters that allow brain cells to communicate, as described in Dr. Russell's Blaylock's book, Excitotoxins: The Taste That Kills. Excitotoxins are exactly what they sound like: Toxins that excite your brain cells to DEATH!

This is a pervasive chemical and is present in many processed foods. You would be quite shocked if you knew how many. It is disguised because food manufacturers are allowed to use substances like yeast extract, gelatin, hydrolyzed protein, and sodium caseinate, which are loaded with excitotoxins and this way they don't have to be declared on the label.

You can review the tables below to see how many hidden sources of MSG there are.[6]

These Ingredients ALWAYS Contain MSG:

MSG	Gelatin	Calcium Caseinate
Monosodium Glutamate	Hydrolyzed Vegetable Protein (HVP)	Textured Protein
Monopotassium Glutamate	Hydrolyzed Plant Protein (HPP)	Yeast Extract
Glutamate	Autolyzed Plant Protein	Yeast food or nutrient
Glutamic Acid	Sodium Caseinate	Autolyzed Yeast

These Ingredients OFTEN Contain MSG:

Malted Barley (flavor)	Flavors, Flavoring	Modified Food Starch
Barley Malt	Reaction Flavors	Rice Syrup or Brown Rice Syrup
Malt Extract or Flavoring	Natural Chicken, Beef or Pork Flavoring or Seasonings	Lipolyzed Butter Fat
Maltodextrin	Soy Sauce or Extract	Low- or No-Fat Items
Caramel Flavoring (coloring)	Soy Protein	Corn Syrup and Corn Syrup Solids
Stock	Soy Protein Isolate or Concentrate	Citric Acid (when processed from corn)
Broth	Cornstarch	Milk Powder
Bouillon	Flowing Agents	Dry Milk Solids

Carrageenan	Wheat, Rice or Oat Protein	Protein-Fortified Milk
Whey Protein	Annatto	Whey Protein Isolate or Concentrate
Products that are Protein-Fortified	Dough Conditioners	Spice
Pectin	Enzyme-modified Products	Gums
Protease and Protease Enzymes	Ultra-Pasteurized Products	Some Fermented Products

The best way to avoid the potential danger of MSG and other food additives is to stay away from them by reducing or eliminating your intake of processed food. To put it simply, your body was designed to eat natural foods as they are found in nature, not artificial substances that are created in a lab.

NOTES

Chapter 4

1 G. Taubes, "What if it's all been a big fat lie?" *New York Times.* 7 July 2002.

2 R. Eli et al. "An adjunctive preventive treatment for cancer: ultraviolet light and ginkgo biloba, together with other antioxidants, are a safe and powerful, but largely ignored, treatment option for the prevention of cancer." *Med Hypotheses* 66, no. 6 (2006): 1152-1156.

3 U. Ravnskov. *The Cholesterol Myths* (New Trends Publishing, 2000), 32-36.

4 G. Zaloga. "Trans fatty acids and coronary heart disease." *Nutr Clin Pract* 21, no. 5 (Oct. 2006): 505-512.

5 A. H. Lichtenstein. "Thematic review series: patient-oriented research. Dietary fat, carbohydrate and protein: effect on plasma lipoprotein patterns". *J Lipid Res* 47, no. 8 (Aug. 2006): 1661-1667.

6 C. N. Bertolino et al. "Dietary trans fatty acid intake and serum lipid profile in Japanese Brazilians in Bauru, Sao Paolo, Brazil." *Cad Saúde Pública* 22, no. 2 (Feb. 2006): 357-364.

7 W. C. Willett. "Trans fatty acids and cardiovascular disease – epidemiological data." *Atheroscl Supplements* 7, no. 2 (May 2006): 5-8.

8   U. Riserus. "Trans fatty acids and insulin resistance." *Atheroscl Supplements* 7, no. 2 (May 2006): 37-39.

9   G. Fernandes. "Dietary lipids and risk of autoimmune disease." *Clin Immunol Immunopathol* 72, no. 2 (Aug. 1994): 193-197.

10   M. T. Salam. "Maternal fish consumption during pregnancy and risk of early childhood asthma." *J Asthma* 42, no. 6 (Jul-Aug. 2005): 513-518.

11   M. C. Morris et al. "Dietary fats and the risk of incident Alzheimer disease." *Arch. Neurol* 60 (2003): 194-200.

12   K. Kuhnt et al. "Dietary supplementation with 11trans- and 12trans-18:1 and oxidative stress in humans." *Am J Clin Nutr* 84, no. 5 (Nov. 2006): 981-8.

13   E. A. Mascioli et al. "Medium chain triglycerides and structured lipids as unique nonglucose energy sources in hyperalimentation." *Lipids* 22, no. 6 (1987): 421.

14   B. O. Barnes and L. Galton, *Hypothyroidism: The Unsuspected Illness.* (New York: Crowell, 1976, and 1994 references).

15   Bruce Fife. "Coconut Oil and Medium-Chain Triglycerides." Coconut Research Center, 2003.

16   M. P. St-Onge et al. "Medium-chain triglycerides increase energy expenditure and decrease adiposity in overweight men." *Obes Res* 11, no. 3 (Mar. 2003): 395-402.

17   S. Sircar. and U. Kansra. "Choice of cooking oils - myths and realities." *J. Indian Med. Assoc* 96, no. 10 (1998): 304

18   T. B. Seaton et al. "Thermic effects of medium-chain and long-chain triglycerides in man." *Am J Clin Nutr* 44 (1986): 630-634.

19   Conrado S. Dayrit. "Coconut Oil in Health and Disease." Philippines Department of Health, 2004.

20   Bruce Fife and Jon Kabara, *The Coconut Oil Miracle*, 4th ed. (Avery, 9 September 2004).

21   Mary Enig. "A New Look At Coconut Oil." Presented at the AVOC Lauric Oils Symposium, Ho Chi Min City, Vietnam, 25 April 1996.

22   Fife and Kabara.

23   Helen Heckler. "Cheap Natural Dry Skin Care Tips for Dry and Damaged Skin." Best Skin Care Tips, 4 April 2007.

24   Fife and Kabara.

25   S. Sierra et al. "Dietary fish oil n-3 fatty acids increase regulatory cytokine production and exert anti-inflammatory effects in two murine models of inflammation." Lipids 41, no. 12 (Dec. 2006): 1115-1125.

26   H. E. Theobald et al. "Low-dose docosahexaenoic acid lowers dias-
      tolic blood pressure in middle-aged men and women." *J Nutr* 137,
      no. 4 (Apr. 2007): 973-978.

27   I. A. Brouwer et al. "N-3 fatty acids, cardiac arrhythmia and fatal
      coronary heart disease." *Prog Lipid Res* 45, no. 4 (Jul. 2006): 357-
      67. Epub 18 Apr. 2006.

28   H. Aarsetoy et al. "Long term influence of regular intake of high
      dose n-3 fatty acids on CD40-ligand, pregnancy-associated
      plasma protein A and matrix metalloproteinase-9 following acute
      myocardial infarction." *Thromb Haemost* 95, no. 2 (Feb. 2006):
      329-336.

29   M. Yokoyama et al. "Effects of eicosapentaenoic acid on major coro-
      nary events in hypercholesterolaemic patients (JELIS): a
      randomised open-label, blinded endpoint analysis." *Lancet* 369, no.
      9567 (31 Mar. 2007): 1090-1098.

30   J. N. Din et al. "Omega-3 fatty acids and cardiovascular disease:
      fishing for a natural treatment." *BMJ* 328, no. 7430 (3 Jan. 2004):
      30-35.

31   N. Kobayashi. "Effect of altering omega-6/omega-3 fatty acid
      ratios on prostate cancer membrane composition, cyclooxygenase-2
      and prostaglandin E2." *Clin Cancer Res* 12, no. 15 (1 Aug. 2006):
      4662-4670.

32   B. Isbilen. "Docosahexanoic acid (omega-3) blocks voltage-gated
      sodium channel activity and migration of MDA-MB-231human
      breast cancer cells." *Int J Biochem Cell Biol* 38, no. 12 (2006: 2173-
      2182.

33   R. S. Chapkin. "Immunomodulatory effects of omega-3 fatty acids:
      putative link to inflammation and colon cancer." *J Nutr* 137. no. 1
      (Jan. 2007): 200S-204S.

34   M. Hashimoto.   "Docosahexanoic acid-induced protective effect
      against impaired learning in amyloid-beta infused rats is associated
      with increased synaptosomal membrane fluidity."   *Clin Exp
      Pharmacol Physiol* 33, no. 10 (Oct. 2006): 934-939.

35   A. P Simopoulos. "Essential fatty acids in health and chronic
      disease." *Am J Clin Nutr* 70, no. 3 (Sept. 1999): 560S-569S.

36   M. F. Leitzmann et al. "Dietary intake of n-3 and n-6 fatty acids
      and the risk of prostate cancer." *Am J Clin Nutr* 80, no. 1 (July
      2004): 204-216.

CHAPTER 5

1   F Vallejo, FA Tomás-Barberán, C García-Viguera, "Phenolic compound contents in edible parts of broccoli inflorescences after domestic cooking," *Journal of the Science of Food Agriculture* 83, no. 14 (2003): 1511-1516.

2   Mark Lucock, "Is folic acid the ultimate functional food component for disease prevention?" *British Medical Journal* 328, no. 7433 (2004): 211.

CHAPTER 6

1   MilkNewsRoom.com. "What America Drinks: How Beverages Relate to Nutrient Intakes and Body Weight." Mary M. Murphy and Judith Spungen Douglass, et al. www.milknewsroom.com /downloads/What_America_Drinks_Report.pdf

2   ScienceBlog.com "Soda, sweet drinks main source of calories in U.S." http://www.scienceblog.com/cms/node/8028

3   DS Ludwig, et al. "Relation between consumption of sugar-sweetened drinks and childhood obesity: a prospective, observational analysis," *The Lancet* 357, no. 9255 (2001): 505-508.

4   U.S. Department of Health and Human Services, Centers for Disease Control and Prevention. "Facts About Chlorine." http://www.bt.cdc.gov/agent/chlorine/basics/facts.asp

5   Washington State Department of Health, Division of Environmental Health, Office of Drinking Water. "Disinfection Byproducts." http://www. doh.wa.gov/ehp/dw/Publications/ disinfection_byproducts.htm

6   Cristina M Villanueva, et al. "Total and specific fluid consumption as determinants of bladder cancer risk," *International Journal of Cancer* 118, no. 8 (2006): 2040-2047.

7   Fluoride Action Network. "HEALTH EFFECTS: Tooth Decay Trends in Fluoridated vs. Unfluoridated Countries" http://fluoridealert.org/health/teeth/caries/who-dmft.html

8   John A Yiamouyiannis. "Water Fluoridation & Tooth Decay: Results from the 1986-1987 National Survey of US Schoolchildren." *Fluoride: Journal of the International Society for Fluoride Research* 23, no. 2 (1990): 55-67.

9   www.organicconsumers.org/articles/article_5499.cfm

10 NTEU CHAPTER 280—U.S. ENVIRONMENTAL PROTECTION AGENCY. "OFFICIAL NTEU CHAPTER 280 POSITION

PAPER ON FLUORIDE" http://nteu280.org/Issues/ Fluoride/ fluoridesummary.htm

11 Earth Policy Institute. "BOTTLED WATER: Pouring Resources Down the Drain." Emily Arnold and Janet Larsen. http://www.earth-policy.org/Updates/2006/Update51.htm

12 http://vitalvotes.com/blogs/public_blog/Our-Oceans-are-Turning-Into-Plastic-18039.aspx#18050

13 Mercola.com "Is Your Bottled Water Really Clean?" www.mercola.com/2003/sep/17/bottled_water.htm

14 William Shotyk and Michael Krachler. "Contamination of Bottled Waters with Antimony Leaching from Polyethylene Terephthalate (PET) Increases upon Storage," *Environmental Science & Technology* 41, no. 5 (2007): 1560-1563.

CHAPTER 7

1 Ma Yunsheng, "Association between Eating Patterns and Obesity in a Free-living US Adult Population," *American Journal of Epidemiology* 158, no. 1 (2003): 85-92.

CHAPTER 10

1 Michael Holick and Mark Jenkins, *The UV Advantage*. (New York: Simon & Schuster, 2003), 52.

2 Gary Null et al. "Death by Medicine." *Life Extension Magazine*, March 2004.

3 F. C. Garland and C. F. Garland. "Occupational sunlight exposure and melanoma in the U.S. Navy." *Archives of Environmental Health* 45, no. 5 (1990): 261-267.

4 V. Bataille et al. "Exposure to the sun and sunbeds and the risk of cutaneous melanoma in the UK: a case-control study." *Eur J Cancer* 40, no. 3 (Feb. 2004): 429-435.

5 V. Bataille et al. "A multicentre epidemiological study on sunbed use and cutaneous melanoma in Europe." *Eur J Cancer* 41, no. 14 (Sept. 2005): 2141-2149.

6 C. F. Garland et al. "Could Sunscreens Increase Melanoma Risk?" *Am J Public Health* 82, no. 4 (1992): 614-615.

7 W.B. Grant. "An estimate of premature cancer mortality in the United States due to inadequate doses of solar ultraviolet-B radiation." *Cancer* 94 (2002): 1867-1875.

8 Based on F. L. Hoffman, *The Mortality of Cancer Throughout the World*. (Prudential Press, 1916), 403-405.

9   Holick and Jenkins, 52.

10   A. R. Webb et al. "Influence of season and latitude on the cutaneous synthesis of vitamin D3: exposure to winter sunlight in Boston and Edmonton will not promote vitamin D3 synthesis in human skin." *J Clin Endocrinol Metab* 67 (1988): 373-378.

11   C. F. Garland et al. "The role of vitamin D in cancer prevention." *Am J Public Health* 96, no. 2 (Feb. 2006): 252-261. Epub 27 Dec. 2005.

12   Ibid.

13   George Wilding and Patrick Remington. "Period Analysis of Prostate Cancer Survival." *Journal of Clinical Oncology* 23, no. 3 (20 January 2005): 407-409.

14   C. F. Garland et al. "Serum 25-hydroxyvitamin D and colon cancer: eight-year prospective study." *Lancet* 2, no. 8673 (18 Nov. 1989): 1176-1178.

15   W.B. Grant. "An estimate of premature cancer mortality in the United States due to inadequate doses of solar ultraviolet-B radiation." *Cancer* 94 (2002): 1867-1875.

16   Marjolein Visser et al. "Low serum concentrations of 25-hydroxyvitamin D in older persons and the risk of nursing home admission." *Am J Clin Nutr* 84 no. 3 (Sept. 2006): 616-622.

17   M. T. Cantorna and B. D. Mahon. "D-hormone and the immune system." *J Rheumatol Suppl* 76 (Sept. 2005): 11-20.

18   Armin Zittermann et al. "Putting cardiovascular disease and vitamin D insufficiency into perspective." *British Journal of Nutrition* 94, no. 4 (Oct. 2005): 483-492.

19   John P. Forman et al. "Vitamin D Intake and Risk of Incident Hypertension: Results From Three Large Prospective Cohort Studies." *Hypertension* 46 (2005): 676.

20   D. S. Grimes DS. "Are statins analogues of vitamin D?" *Lancet* 368, no. 9529 (1 July 2006): 83-86.

21   M. S. Saporito et al. "Pharmacological induction of nerve growth factor mRNA in adult rat brain." *Exp Neurol* 123, no. 2 (Oct. 1993): 295-302.

22   K. Kinuta et al. "Vitamin D is an important factor in estrogen biosynthesis of both female and male gonads." *Endocrinology* 141 (2000): 1317-1324.

23   K. V. Luong and L. T. Nguyen. "Vitamin D and cardiovascular disease." *Curr Med Chem* 13, no. 20 (2006): 2443-2447.

24 Y. Sato et al. "Low-dose vitamin D prevents muscular atrophy and reduces falls and hip fractures in women after stroke: a randomized controlled trial." *Cerebrovasc Dis* 20, no. 3 (2005):187-192. Epub 27 July 2005.

25 Richard Hobday, *The Healing Sun*. (Scotland: Findhorn Press, 1999), 18.

26 B. R. East. "Mean Annual Hours of Sunshine and the Incidence of Dental Caries." *Am J Public Health* 29 (1939): 777-780.

27 M C. Chapuy et al. "Vitamin D3 and Calcium to Prevent Hip Fractures in Elderly Women." *NEJM* 327 (1992): 1637-1642.

28 Encyclopedia Britannica, Inc. "Medicine: Timeline of Achievements." In *Britannica Guide to the Nobel Prizes*. Encyclopedia Britannica, Inc., 1997.

29 J. J. Cannell et al. "Epidemic influenza and vitamin D." *Epidemiology and Infection* 136 (Dec. 2006): 1129-1140.

30 Ibid.

31 R. E. Hope-Simpson. "Age And Secular Distributions Of Virus-Proven Influenza Patients In Successive Epidemics 1961-1976 In Cirencester: Epidemiological Significance Discussed." *J Hyg (Lond)* 92, no. 3 (Jun. 1984): 303-336.

32 E. Kamycheva et al. "Intakes of Calcium and Vitamin D Predict Body Mass Index in the Population of Northern Norway." *J Nutr* 132 (2002): 102-106.

33 H. Shi et al. "1alpha,25-Dihydroxyvitamin D3 modulates human adipocyte metabolism via nongenomic action." *FASEB J* 15, no. 14 (Dec. 2001): 2751-2753.

34 Lisa A Houghton and Reinhold Vieth. "The case against ergocalciferol (vitamin D2) as a vitamin supplement." *Am J Clin Nutr* 84, no. 4 (Oct. 2006): 694-697.

35 A. F. Hess et al. "Newer aspects of the therapeutics of viosterol (irradiated ergosterol)." *JAMA* 94 (1930): 1885.

36 E. Hypponen. "Intake of vitamin D and risk of type 1 diabetes: a birth-cohort study." *Lancet* 358, no. 9292 (3 Nov. 2001): 1500-1503.

37 International Society for Developmental Neuroscience meeting in Sydney, Australia (Feb. 2002).

38 S. R. Kreiter et al. "Nutritional rickets in African American breast-fed infants." *J. Pediatr* 137 (2000): 153-157.

39 N. A. Badian. "Reading disability in an epidemiological context incidence and environmental correlates." *J Learn Disabil* 17, no. 3 (Mar. 1984): 129-136.

40   A. Becker et al. "Transient prenatal vitamin D deficiency is associated with subtle alterations in learning and memory functions in adult rats." *Behav Brain Res* 161, no. 2 (20 Jun. 2005): 306-312.

41   Eva S. Schernhammer et al. "Rotating Night Shifts and Risk of Breast Cancer in Women Participating in the Nurses' Health Study." *J Nat Cancer Inst* 93, no. 20 (2001): 1563-1568.

42   U.S. Environmental Protection Agency, *Evaluation of the Potential Carcinogenicity of Electromagnetic Fields (External Review Draft).* (Washington, DC: US Environmental Protection Agency Office of Research and Development, National Center for Environmental Assessment, Washington Office, March 1990).

43   Shamas T. Butt and Terje Christensen. *Radiat. Prot. Dosimetry* 91 (2000): 83.

44   Ibid.

45   Jo Reville. "Sunscreen is No Protection Against Cancer." *The Guardian.* 28 Sept. 2003.

CHAPTER 11

1   Cristina Fortes, "Depressive Symptoms Lead to Impaired Cellular Immune Response," *Psychotherapy and Psychosomatics* 72, no. 5 (2003): 253-260.

2   Tim Smith, professor, psychology, University of Utah, Salt Lake City (American Psychosomatic meeting, Denver, Colorado, March 3, 2006).

3   Janice K. Kiecolt-Glaser, et al., "Hostile Marital Interactions, Proinflammatory Cytokine Production, and Wound Healing," *Archives of General Psychiatry* 62, no. 12 (2005): 1377-1384.

4   T. Maruta, et al., "Optimism-pessimism assessed in the 1960s and self-reported health status 30 years later," *Mayo Clinic Proceedings* 77, no. 8 (2002): 748-753.

5   Glenn V. Ostir, "Hypertension in Older Adults and the Role of Positive Emotions," *Psychosomatic Medicine* 68, no. 5 (2006): 727-733.

6   R.J. Davidson, et al., "Alterations in brain and immune function produced by mindfulness meditation," *Psychosomatic Medicine* 65, no. 4 (2003): 564-7 Louise Hay, *Heal Your Body* (Carlsbad: Hay House, Inc., 1982).

7   Louise Hay, *Heal Your Body* (Carlsbad: Hay House, Inc., 1982).

CHAPTER 12

1   T. G. Pickering et al. "Could hypertension be a consequence of the 24/7 society? The effects of sleep deprivation and shift work." Journal of Clinical Hypertension 8, No. 11 (Nov. 2006): 819-822.

2   D. F. Kripke et al. "Mortality associates with sleep duration and insomnia". Arch Gen Psych 59 (2002): 131-136.

3   C. E. Wright et al. "Poor sleep the night before an experimental stressor predicts reduced NK cell mobilization and slowed recovery in healthy women." Brain Behav Immun 21, no. 3 (Mar. 2007): 358-363.

4   N. T. Ayas et al. "A prospective study of sleep duration and coronary heart disease in women." Arch Internal Med 163 (2003): 205-209.

5   T. G. Pickering et al. "Could hypertension be a consequence of the 24/7 society? The effects of sleep deprivation and shift work." Journal of Clinical Hypertension 8, No. 11 (Nov. 2006): 819-822.

6   N. T. Ayas et al. "A prospective study of self-reported sleep duration and incident diabetes in women." Diabetes Care 26 (Feb. 2003); 380-384.

7   H. K. Yaggi et al. "Sleep duration as a risk factor for the development of type 2 diabetes." Diabetes Care 29 (2006): 657-661.

8   K. Spiegel et al. "Impact of sleep debt on metabolic and endocrine function." Lancet 354, no. 9188 (23 Oct. 1999): 1435-1439.

9   G. Cizza et al. "A link between short sleep and obesity: building the evidence for causation". Sleep 28 (2005): 1217-1220.

10 Cherie Calbom and John Calbom. Sleep Away The Pounds: Optimize Your Sleep and Reset Your Metabolism for Maximum Weight Loss (Warner Wellness, 2007).

11 V. Roman et al. "Differential effects of chronic partial sleep deprivation and stress on Serotonin-1A and muscarinic acetylcholine receptor sensitivity". Journal of Sleep Research 15, no. 4 (Dec. 2006):386-94

12 C. P. Landrigan et al. "Effect of reducing interns' work hours on serious medical errors in intensive care units." N Engl J Med 351 (2004): 1838-1848.

13 S. Sephton et al. "Circadian disruption in cancer: a neuroendocrine-immune pathway from stress to disease?" Brain Behav Immun 5 (2003): 321-328.

14 S.C. Larsson et al. "Dietary carbohydrate, glycemic index and glycemic load in relation to risk of colorectal cancer in women." Am J Epidemiol 165, no. 3 (1 Feb. 2007): 256-261.

15   T. A. Wehr. "Melatonin and seasonal rhythms." J Biol Rhythms 12, no. 6 (Dec. 1997): 518-527.

16   M. Tuzcu et al. "Effect of melatonin and vitamin E on diabetes-induced learning and memory impairment in rats." Eur J Pharmacol 537, nos. 1-3 (10 May 2006): 106-110.

17   A. N. Vgontzas et al. "Chronic insomnia is associated with nytohe-meral activation of the hypothalamic-pituitary-adrenal axis: clinical implications." Journal of Clinical Endocrinology and Metabolism 96, no.8 (Aug. 2001): 3787-3794.

18   R. J. Raymann et al. "Skin temperature and sleep-onset latency: changes with age and insomnia." Physiol. Behav 90, no. 2-3 (2007): 257-266.

19   E. Hartmann "L-tryptophan: a rational hypnotic with clinical potential." Am J. Psychiatry 134, no. 4 (Apr. 1977): 366-370.

20   O. Bruni et al. "L-5-hydroxytryptophan treatment of sleep terrors in children." Eur J Pediatr 163, no. 7 (July 2004): 402-407.

CHAPTER 13

1   W. Duke. "Saccharin: A Real Look at an Artificial Sweetener," web1.caryacademy.org.

2   W. Brody. "Biomedical Engineering Lecture Series: From Minds to Minefields: Negotiating the Demilitarized Zone Between Industry and Academia," 1999.

3   P. Macinnis, P. Bittersweet: The Story of Sugar. (Crows Nest: Allen & Unwin, 2002).

4   M. W. Wagner. "Cyclamate Acceptance." Science 168 (1970): 1605.

5   J. M. Taylor, M. A. Weinberger, and L. Friedman. "Chronic Toxicity and Carcinogenicity to the Urinary Bladder of Sodium Saccharin in the In Utero-Exposed Rat," Toxicology and Applied Pharmacology 1, no. 54 (June 1980): 57–75.

6   R. A. Squire. "Histopathological Evaluation of Rat Urinary Bladders from the IRDC Two-Generation Bioassay of Sodium Saccharin," Food and Chemical Toxicology 23, nos. 4–5 (Apr.–May 1985): 491–497.

7   S. Fukushima et al. "Differences in Susceptibility to Sodium Saccharin Among Various Strains of Rats and Other Animal Species," Gann 74 (Feb. 1983): 8–20.

8   W. Duke. "Saccharin: A Real Look at an Artificial Sweetener," web1.caryacademy.org.

NOTES

9   R. Powelson. "Warnings No Longer Required for Products Containing Saccharin." *Nando Media* (Jan. 2001, April. 2001), www.nandotimes.com.

10   H. J. Roberts, *Aspartame Disease: An Ignored Epidemic* (West Palm Beach: Sunshine Sentinel Press, 2001).

11   Cori Brackett and J. T. Waldron. *Sweet Misery: A Poisoned World* (Sound and Fury Productions, 2004).

12   Study E-33, 34, Cross Reference E-87, Master File 134 for Aspartame, FDA Hearing Clerk's Office.

13   Special Investigation, *Common Cause* 10, no. 4 (July/August 1984).

14   J. Turner. *The Aspartame/Nutrasweet Fiasco*, www. stevia.net/aspartame.htm.

15   Brackett and Waldron.

16   "Preapproval, 'Research' & History of Aspartame", www. holisticmed.com/aspartame/history.faq.

17   J. Bressler et al. "FDA Report on Searle," August 4, 1977, www.dorway.com/bressler.txt.

18   A. Constantine. "History of Aspartame," 2004, www. wnho.net/history_of_aspartame.htm.

19   Brackett and Waldron.

20   Ibid.

21   A. Constantine. "History of Aspartame," 2004, www. wnho.net/history_of_aspartame.htm.

22   U.S. General Accounting Office, "Briefing Report to the Honorable Howard Metzenbaum, U.S. Senate; Food and Drug Administraion, Six Former HHS Employees' Involvement In Aspartame's Approval," GAO/HRD-86-109BR, July 1986.

23   Roberts.

24   Russell Blaylock, *Excitotoxins: The Taste That Kills.* (New Mexico: MD Health Press, 1996).

25   R. G. Walton, "Seizure and Mania after High Intake of Aspartame," *Psychosomatics* 27, no. 3 (March 1986): 218, 220.

26   W. M. Pardridge, "The Safety of Aspartame," *Journal of the American Medical Association* 256, no. 19 (November 21, 1986): 267.

27   J. W. Olney, L. G. Sharpe, and R. D. Feigin, "Glutamate Induced Brain Damage in Infant Primates," *Journal of Neuropathology and Experimental Neurology* 31 (1972): 464–88.

28   Betty Martini. "Interview with Dr. Roberts," 1998, www.dorway.com/hjrinv.txt.

29   O. M. Sejersted et al. "Formate Concentrations in Plasma from Patients Poisoned with Methanol." *Acta Medica Scandinavica* 213 (1983): 105–10.

30   J. Bowen. "Aspartame Toxicity and Methanol, Ethanol, Pectin, Methyl Alcohol," www.321recipes.com.

31   H. O. Adami, L. B. Signorello, and D. Trichopoulos, "Towards an Understanding of Breast Cancer Etiology," *Seminars in Cancer Biology* 8 (1998): 255–62.

32   References listed are available at the end of the following Web page: www.holisticmed.com/aspartame/scf2002-response.htm. Other reviews on formaldehyde can be found at www. drthrasher .org/research.html. Studies cited:

      J. Shaham et al. "DNA—protein Crosslinks, a Biomarker of Exposure to Formaldehyde—in vitro and in vivo Studies," Carcinogenesis 17, no. 1 (1996): 121–125.

      D. M Main and T.J. Hogan "Health Effect of Low-Level Exposure to Formaldehyde," *Journal of Occupational Medicine* 25 (1983): 896-900.

      Kai-Shen Liu et al. "Irritant Effects of Formaldehyde Exposure in Mobile Homes," *Environmental Health Perspectives* 94 (1993): 91-94.

      A. K. Srivastava et al. "Clinical studies of employees in a sheet-form-ing process at a paper mill," *Veterinary and Human Toxicology* 34, no. 6 (1992): 525–527.

      S. Burdach and K. Wechselberg. "Damages to health in schoos. Complaints caused by the use of formaldehyde-emitting materials in school buildings," *Fortschritte Med* 98, no. 11 (1980): 379-384.

      K. H. Kilburn. "Indoor air effects after building renovation and in man¬ufactured homes," *American Journal of Medical Science* 320, no. 4 (2000): 249-254.

      K. H. Kilburn. "Neurobehavioral impairment and seizures from formaldehyde," *Archives of Environmental Health* 49, no. 1 (1994): 37-44.

      L. Proietti et al. "Occupational exposure to formaldehyde at a service of pathologic anatomy," *Giornale Italiano di Medicina del Lavoro ed Ergonomia* 24, no. 1 (2002): 32-34.

      K. H. Kilburn et al. "Neurobehavioral and respi¬ratory symptoms of formaldehyde and xylene exposure in histology techni-cians," *Archives of Environmental Health* 40, no. 4 (1985): 229-233.

33   National Cancer Institute SEER Program Data, K. E. Jellinger et al.,
      "Primary Central Nervous System Lymphomas: An Update,"
      Journal of the National Cancer Institute 84 (1992): 414–422.

34   J. G. Gurney, J. M. Pogoda, and E. A. Holly, "Aspartame
      Consumption in Relation to Childhood Brain Tumor Risk: Results
      from a Case-Control Study," *Journal of the National Cancer
      Institute* 89 (1997): 1072–1074.

35   Study E33-34 in Master File 134 on aspartame, on file at the FDA
      Hearing Clerk's Office 2001.

36   M. Soffritti et al., "First Experimental Demonstration of the
      Multipotential Carcinogenic Effects of Aspartame Administered in
      the Feed to Sprague-Dawley Rats," *Environmental Health
      Perspectives* 114, no. 3 (March 2006): 379–85.

37   "Aspartame and the FDA" (April 20, 1995), presidiotex.com/
      aspartame/Facts/Aspartame_and_the_FDA/aspartame_and_the_f
      da.html.

38   F. Graves,"Results of *Common Cause* Magazine Investigation of
      FDA's Approval of Aspartame," July 1984.

39   "Morbidity and Mortality Weekly Report," www.cdc.gov.

40   M. Jacobson, "Artificial Sweetener 'Sunett' Should Not Be Used in
      Diet Soda, New Tests Needed, Cancer Experts Tell FDA," 1996,
      <www.cspinet.org/new/ask.html.com> (26 June 2006). Sample
      quotes from cancer experts' letters on acesulfame testing,
      www.cspinet.org/foodsafety/additives_acesulfame.html.

41   "Sugar Substitutes—Are They Safe?" ag.arizona.edu.

42   "The Secret Dangers of Splenda (Sucralose), an Artificial Sweetener,"
      www.mercola.com/2000/dec/3/sucralose_dangers.htm.

43   Elizabeth Esfahani, "Finding the Sweet Spot," 1 November 2005,
      money.cnn.com/magazines/business2/business2_archive/2005/1
      1/01/8362835/index.htm.

44   Burkhard Bilger, "The Search for Sweet," *New Yorker*, 22 May
      2006.

45   H. C. Grice and L. A. Goldsmith, "Sucralose—An Overview of the
      Toxicity Data," Food and Chemical Toxicology 38 (2000): S1–S6.

46   Global Strategic Management Splenda Paper,
      plaza.ufl.edu/mr2/MAN6636/splendaPaper.doc.

47   Melanie Warner, "US: Senomyx's Fake Flavors," New York Times, 6
      April 2005, http>//www.corpwatch.org/article.php?id=12053.

48   Anonymous source.

49   Interview with two food industry insiders who wish to remain
      anonymous.

NOTES

50   21 CFR Part 172 [Docket NO. 87F-0086 Food Additives Permitted for Direct Addition to Food for Human Consumptions; Sucralose]. Study E051.

51   S. W. Mann et al., "A Carcinogenicity Study of Sucralose in the CD-1 Mouse," *Food and Chemical Toxicology* 38, suppl. 2 (2000): S91-7.

52   Chemical Abstracts Service Registry num¬ber for sucralose: 56038-13-2, www.cas.org; www.SweetDeception.com/Patent.

53   "Highly Hazardous Chemicals", <www.ehs. psu.edu/hazmat/highly_hazardous_chemicals. pdf>.

54   "Frequently Asked Questions about SPLENDA® Brand Sweetener," www. splenda.com.

55   James Bowen, "The Lethal Science of Splenda, A Poisonous Chlorocarbon," May 2005, www.wnho.net /splenda_chloro-carbon.htm.

56   Kevin Ban, "Toxicity, Hydrocarbon Insecticides," emedicine.com, December 2005, <www.emedicine.com/emerg/topic255. htm>.

57   "The Science of Splenda Brand Sweetener (Sucralose)," www.Splenda.com,www.splendaprofessional. com.

58   Stuart Graham, Additives Evaluation Branch (H FF-158), Department of Health & Human Services To Ms. Blondell Anderson Through: G.N. Biddle, PhD, Memorandum, 8 August 1991, Subject: Sucralose—Final Review and Evaluation FOOD ADDITIVE PETITION NO. 7A3987, Washington, D.C., 21.

59   Studies cited:

"1,6-dichloro-1, 6-dideoxyfructose: Investigation of Effects on Bone Marrow Chromosomes of the Rat after Acute and Subacute Oral Administration," EO19.

"1,6–dichloro-l ,6-dideoxyfructose: Assessment of Its Mutagenic Potential in Histidine Auxotrophs of Salmonella typhimurium," E020.

"1,6-dichloro-l,6-dideoxyfructose: Assessment of Its Mutagenic Potential in Drosophila melanoqaster, Using the Sex-Linked Recessive Lethal Test," E021.

"Evaluation of Test Article 1,6-dichlorofructose (MRI #536) for Mutagenic Potential Employing the L5178Y TK+/ Mutagenesis Assay," E022.

"Salmonella/Mammalian Microsome Plate Incorporation Mutagenesis Assay," E023.

"Evaluation of Test Article 1, 6-dichlorofructose (MRI #629) for Mutagenic Potential EmDloying the L5178Y TK+/ Mutagenesis Assay," E024.

FDA studies labeled as E148, E054, E052, E032, E053.

60   "1,6-Dichloro-1,6-dideoxyfructose: Metabolism in the Rat." Study E147. Laboratory: Department of Biochemistry, University College, Wales, UK, 8 March 1988, File location: FAP 7A3987, vol. 98, A002598-02661.

61   Jacobson, Michael. "Splenda Should Stop Confusing Consumers, Says CSPI" CSPI *Newsroom*. cspinet.org/new/ 200502141.html.

62   "Cost Is the Key to Neotame's Success," Food Navigator-USA.com, 2005, www.foodnavigator-usa.com/news-by-product/news.asp?id=58489&idCat=88&k=cost-is-the.

63   D. Richard, *Stevia Rebaudiana: Nature's Sweet Secret* (CITY: Vital Health Publishing, 1996).

64   Fujita and Tomoyoshi, "Safety and Utilization of Stevia Sweetener."

65   L. N. Chen and E. S. Parham, "College Students' Use of High-Intensity Sweeteners Is Not Consistently Associated with Sugar Consumption," *Journal of the American Dietetic Association* 91 (1991): 686–90.

66   "U.S. Study Links Diet Pop to Obesity," 15 June 2005, www.ctv.ca/servlet/ArticleNews/story/CTVNews/11188405854 67_33/?hub=TopStories.

67   FDA, "A Food Labeling Guide—Appendix A: Definitions of Nutrient Content Claims," www.cfsan.fda.gov/~dms/flg-6a.html.

68   Richard Bernstein, *Dr. Bernstein's Diabetes Solution* (Boston: Little, Brown and Company, 2003), 138, emphasis added.

CHAPTER 14

1   U.S. Department of Agriculture Release No. 0306.06, "Genetically Engineered Rice." U.S. Department of Agriculture. www.usda.gov/wps/portal/usdahome?contentidonly=true&contentid=2006/08/0306.xml

2   The Pew Initiative on Food and Biotechnology. "Public Sentiment About Genetically Modified Food (December 2006 update)." University of Richmond. pewagbiotech.org/polls/

3   "Global Seed Industry Concentration—2005," *ETC Group Communiqué*, September/October 2005, Issue 90.

4   "Oligopoly, Inc. 2005 Concentration in Corporate Power," ETC Group Communiqué, November/December 2005, Issue 91.

5   E.S. Dennis, R.I.S. Brettell and W.J Peacock, "A tissue culture induced Adh2 null mutant of maize results from a single base change," Molecular & General Genetics 210, no. 1 (1987): 181-183; and R.I.S. Brettell, et al., "Molecular analysis of a somaclonal mutant of maize alcohol dehydrogenase," *Molecular & General Genetics* 202, no. 2 (1986): 235-239.

6   NRC/IOM: Committee on Identifying and Assessing Unintended Effects of Genetically Engineered Foods on Human Health, *Safety of Genetically Engineered Foods: Approaches to assessing unintended health effects* (Washington D.C: The National Academies Press, 2004); and D.A. Kessler, et al., "The safety of foods developed by biotechnology," *Science* 256 (1992): 1747-1832.

7   Jeffrey Smith, "Genetically Modified Corn Study Reveals Health Damage and Cover-up, Spilling the Beans." Institute for Responsible Technology. www.responsibletechnology.org

8   M.A. Noble, P.D. Riben and G.J. Cook, "Microbiological and epidemiological surveillance program to monitor the health effects of Foray 48B BTK spray." (Report to Vancouver, B.C. Ministry of Forests, Province of British Columbia, September 30, 1992).

9   J.R. Samples and H. Buettner, "Ocular infection caused by a biological insecticide," *The Journal of Infectious Diseases* 148, no. 3 (1983): 614 (as reported in: Carrie Swadener, "Bacillus thuringiensis (B.t.)," *Journal of Pesticide Reform* 14, no. 3 (1994).)

10 M. Green, et al., "Public health implications of the microbial pesticide Bacillus thuringiensis: An epidemiological study, Oregon, 1985-86," *American Journal of Public Health* 80, no. 7 (1990): 848-852.

11 GMWatch.org. "Mortality in Sheep Flocks after Grazing on Bt Cotton Fields—Warangal District, Andhra Pradesh, Report of the Preliminary Assessment April 2006." www.gm-watch.org/archive2.asp?arcid=6494

12 "Monsanto Cited In Crop Losses," *NYTimes.com*, June 16, 1998 , query.nytimes.com/gst/fullpage.html?res=9A04EED6153DF935 A25755C0A96E958260; and Greenpeace.org. "Genetic instability and crop failures." archive.greenpeace.org/geneng/reports/gmo/intrgmo5.htm

13 Antje Lorch, "Monsanto Bribes in Indonesia, Monsanto Fined For Bribing Indonesian Officials to Avoid Environmental Studies for Bt Cotton." Mindfully.org. www.mindfully.org/GE/2005/Monsanto-Bribes-Indonesia1sep05.htm

14   Centre for Sustainable Agriculture. "Bt Cottonz—No Respite for Andhra Pradesh Farmers More than 400 crores' worth losses for Bt Cotton farmers in Kharif, 2005." GMWatch.org www.gmwatch.org/archive2.asp?arcid=6393; see also November 14, 2005 article in www.NewKerala.com regarding Madhya Pradesh.

15   Abdul Qayum and Kiran Sakkhari, "Did Bt Cotton Save Farmers in Warangal? A season long impact study of Bt Cotton - Kharif 2002 in Warangal District of Andhra Pradesh?" (AP Coalition in Defence of Diversity & Deccan Development Society, Hyderabad, 2003).

16   Netherwood, et al., "Assessing the survival of transgenic plant DNA in the human gastrointestinal tract," *Nature Biotechnology* 22, no. 2 (2004).

17   Sophie Richard et al., "Differential Effects of Glyphosate and Roundup on Human Placental Cells and Aromatase," Environmental Health Perspectives 113, no. 6 (2005).

18   Mark Townsend, "Why soya is a hidden destroyer," *Daily Express*, March 12, 1999.

19   G. A. Kleter and A. A. C. M. Peijnenburg, "Screening of transgenic proteins expressed in transgenic food crops for the presence of short amino acid sequences indentical to potential, IgE-binding linear epitopes of allergens," *BMC Structural Biology* 2 (2002): 8-19.

20   S.W.B. Ewen and A. Pusztai, "Effects of diets containing genetically modified potatoes expressing Galanthus nivalis lectin on rat small intestine," *Lancet* 354 (1999): 1727-1728.

21   Ian F. Pryme and Rolf Lembcke, "In Vivo Studies on Possible Health Consequences of Genetically Modified Food and Feed—with Particular Regard to Ingredients Consisting of Genetically Modified Plan Materials," *Nutrition and Health* 17 (2003): 1-8.

22   Jeffrey M. Smith, *Seeds of Deception* (Iowa: Yes! Books, 2003).

23   A. Pusztai, et al., "Genetically Modified Foods: Potential Human Health Effects," (In: JPF D'Mello, ed., *Food Safety: Contaminants and Toxins* (Wallingford Oxon, UK: CAB International Publishing, 2003).

24   Craig Canine, "Hear No Evil: In its determination to become a model corporate citizen, is the FDA ignoring potential dangers in the nation's food supply?" *Eating Well*, July/August 1991.

25   Jeffrey M. Smith, *Seeds of Deception* (Iowa: Yes! Books, 2003).

26   GM Nation? "GM Nation? The findings of the public debate." www.gmnation.org.uk/ut_09/ut_9_6.htm#summary

27   The Natural Marketing Institute, "Hot New Consumer and Retail Trends" (Presented at Expo West, March 24, 2006).

CHAPTER 15

1.   E.T. Horn Company FoodTech Group. "E.T. Horn Company Selected By Cargill Foods as Exclusive Distributor of Lecithin Products in Western States." E.T. Horn Company. www.ethorn.com/foodtech/news_item_20040625.htm

2.   Srikanth Yellayi, "The phytoestrogen genistein induces thymic and immune changes: A human health concern?" *Proceedings of the National Academy of Sciences* 99, no. 11 (2002): 7616-7621.

3.   L.R. White, et al., "Association of mid-life consumption of tofu with late life cognitive impairment and dementia: the Honolulu-Asia Aging Study" (Fifth International Conference on Alzheimer's Disease, #487, Osaka, Japan, July 27, 1996).

4.   L.R. White, et al., "Brain aging and midlife tofu consumption," *Journal of the American College of Nutrition* 19, no. 2 (2000): 242-55.

CHAPTER 16

1   R.S. Mendelsohn, *Confessions of a Medical Heretic* (Chicago: Warner Books, 1979).

2   Deborah A. Gust, et al., "Parent Attitudes Toward Immunizations and Healthcare Providers," *American Journal of Preventive Medicine* 29, no. 2 (2005): 105-112.

3   SP Calandrillo, "Vanishing vaccinations: why are so many Americans opting out of vaccinating their children?" *University of Michigan Journal of Law Reform* 37, no. 2 (2004): 353-440.

4   Centers for Disease Control and Prevention. " 2007 Childhood & Adolescent Immunization Schedules." National Immunization Program. www.cdc.gov/nip/recs/child-schedule.htm#printable (accessed February 28, 2007).

5   NewsWithViews.com. "Why You Should Avoid Taking Vaccines." James Howenstine. www.newswithviews.com/Howenstine/james.htm (accessed February 28, 2007).

6   I. Golden, *Vaccination & Homoeoprophylaxis? A Review of Risks and Alternatives* (Gisborne, Victoria, Australia: Isaac Golden Publications, 2005).

7   The National Health and Medical Research Council, *The Australian Immunisation Handbook* (2003)

8   L. Gustafsson, et al., "A Controlled Trial of a Two-Component Acellular, a Five-Component Acellular, and a Whole-Cell Pertussis Vaccine," *New England Journal of Medicine* 334, no. 6 (1996):349-356.

9   A. Puri, et al., "Measles Vaccine Efficacy Evaluated by Case Reference Technique," *Indian Pediatrics* 39 (2002): 556-560.

10   The National Health and Medical Research Council, *The Australian Immunisation Handbook* (2003)

11   The National Health and Medical Research Council, The Australian Immunisation Handbook (2003)

12   J. Cherry, et al., "Report of the Task Force on Pertussis and Pertussis Immunization," *Pediatrics* 81, no. 6 (1988): 972, 973.

13   M. Odent et al., "Pertussis vaccination and asthma: Is there a link?" *Journal of the American Medical Association* 272, no. 8 (1994): 592-3.
     Odent M et al, (1994b) *Pertussis Vaccination and Asthma: Is There a Link?* British Medical Journal, Vol 272; pp. 592-3.

14   T. Kemp, et al., "Is infant immunization a risk factor for childhood asthma or allergy?" *Epidemiology* 8, no. 6 (1997): 678-80.

15   I. Golden, *Homoeoprophylaxis—A Fifteen-Year Clinical Study* (Gisborne, Victoria, Australia: Isaac Golden Publications, 2004).

16   (a) A.J. Wakefield, et al, "Ileal-lymphoid nodular hyperplasia, non-specific colitis, and pervasive developmental disorder in children," *Lancet* 351, no. 9103 (1998): 637-641.
     (b) A.J. Wakefield and S.M. Montgomery, "Measles, mumps, rubella vaccine: through a glass, darkly," *Adverse Drug Reactions and Toxicological Reviews* 19, no. 4 (2000): 265-283.

17   V. Singh and V. Yang, "Serological association of measles virus and human herpes virus-6 with brain antibodies in autism," *Clinical Immunology and Immunopathology* 88, no. 1 (1998): 105-108.

18   Centers for Disease Control and Prevention. "Prevalence of Autism Spectrum Disorders, Autism and Developmental Disabilities Monitoring Network, 14 Sites, United States, 2002." Morbidity and Mortality Weekly Report February 9, 2007 www.cdc.gov/mmwr/preview/mmwrhtml/ss5601a2.htm (accessed February 28, 2007).

19   Mercola.com "Mercury Contributes To Alzheimer's Disease." www.mercola.com/2001/apr/7/alzheimers_mercury.htm

20   Mercola.com "Alzheimer's Vaccine Causes Life-Threatening Side Effects" www.mercola.com/2003/apr/5/alzheimers_vaccine.htm

21 Institute of Medicine, *Adverse Effects of Pertussis and Rubella Vaccines* (Washington, DC: National Academy Press, 1991).

22 Mercola.com "Sugar Increases Polio Risk—Lessons For Other Viral Infections" www.Mercola.com/article/sugar/polio_sugar.htm

23 Mercola.com "How To Legally Avoid Unwanted Immunizations Of All Kinds." www.Mercola.com/article/vaccines/legally_avoid _shots.htm

CHAPTER 17

1 David Steinman and Samuel Epstein, *The Safe Shopper's Bible*. Macmillan, New York: 1995: 2-4.

2 Ibid., 4.

3 Ibid., 2.

4 Kim Erickson, *Drop-Dead Gorgeous*. McGraw- Hill, New York: 2002: 19–20.

5 Steinman and Epstein, 2–4.

6 Erickson, 9-10.

7 Pratima Raichur, *Absolute Beauty*, HarperCollins, New York: 1997: 100.

8 Caroline Gorman and Marie Hyde Dickson, *Less Toxic Alternatives*, Optimum, Texas: 1997.

9 B.C.Wolverton, *How to Grow Fresh Air*. Penguin Group, New York: 1996: 8-13.

10 Ibid., 22–23, 40.

11 Steinman and Epstein, 73.

12 Gorman and Dickson.

13 Erickson, 20, 28.

14 Gorman and Dickson.

15 Steinman and Epstein, 253.

16 Gorman and Dickson.

17 Steinman and Epstein, 201–218.

18 Gorman and Dickson.

19 Steinman and Epstein, 240–241

20 Gorman and Dickson.

21 Pierre Jean Cousin, *Facelift at Your Fingertips*. Storey Books, Vermont: 2000, 22-24.

CHAPTER 18

1 Daniel S. Budnitz, et al., "National Surveillance of Emergency Department Visits for Outpatient Adverse Drug Events," *Journal of the American Medical Association* 296, no. 15 (2006): 1858-1866.

2 C. Neurath, "Tooth decay trends for 12 year olds in nonfluoridated and fluoridated countries," *Fluoride* 38, no. 4 (2005): 324-325.

3 F. Vallejo, F.A. Tomás-Barberán and C. García-Viguera, "Phenolic compound contents in edible parts of broccoli inflorescences after domestic cooking," *Journal of the Science of Food and Agriculture* 83, no. 14 (2003): 1511-1516.

4 Arnold Schecter et al., "Human Consumption of Methyleugenol and Its Elimination from Serum," *Environmental Health Perspectives* 112, no. 6 (2004): 678.

5 James P. Maloney, et al., "Systemic Absorption of Food Dye in Patients with Sepsis," *New England Journal of Medicine* 343, no. 14 (2000): 1047-1048.

6 Debby Anglesey, *Battling the MSG Myth* (Front Porch Productions, 2007) and MSGMyth.com. "Hidden Names for MSG." www.msgmyth.com

APPENDIX A
How To Legally Avoid
Unwanted Vaccinations

As you read this work and put its principles into practice, there are two basic axioms you never want to forget. They are the rock upon which all your actions are based.

1. Nobody, anywhere or at any time and under any circumstances, has the right or power in this country to immunize you or your children against your will and conviction. If they attempt to do so, you can legally charge them with "assault with a deadly weapon" and have the full resources of our laws behind you.

2. At all times in attempting to avoid unwanted immunization, you have the Law of the Land behind you. Those who would try to vaccinate you against your will are on very shaky ground. Into every compulsory immunization law in America are written legal exceptions and waivers which are there specifically to protect you from the attempted tyranny of officialdom. It is not only your right, but your obligation to use them, if this is what your conscience tells you.

APPENDIX A

Article 1

In all your contact with any members of the school, public health, or legal establishment, always remain calm, courteous, and humbly reverent toward their position. You are only asking of them that which the law duly binds them to give you. There is no reason, or advantage, to be gained by antagonizing them.

Most of these officials believe they are discharging their trust as outlined by law. If they are overstepping the law, then you must very diplomatically bring the true facts to their attention, but without attempting to belittle them.

The more you can preserve their ego, the more easily and quickly you are likely to get what you desire—a waiver of immunization.

Rule No. 1: Do not harass, belittle, or antagonize officials unnecessarily.

Article 2

All compulsory laws concerning vaccination (including the military) contain exceptions and waivers. It is these protections placed in the laws that you may legally use to exclude yourself and your children. Surprisingly, these exceptions were placed there, not for your sake (although you may take advantage of them), but for the protection of the establishment.

How is this? Let us assume that these exceptions were not there and everyone was actually forced to be immunized. Should a child die or become mentally or physically disabled, the parent would have the perfect case to sue the doctor, the school, the health department, and even the state legislature for enormous damages.

Since they allowed no exceptions, they must accept full responsibility for all the adverse consequences of the law.

However, if exception waivers are placed in the law, the responsibility is then transferred back to the parent. If a child should be injured by immunization, the officials can say, "Well, the parent should have exempted him if they thought there was any danger."

Therefore, there is, in truth, no such thing as a compulsory vaccination law in this country. They are **ALL**, in essence, **voluntary**. The problem is that practically no one in authority will let you know this fact.

Rule No. 2: There are no compulsory vaccination laws. All are voluntary, and you are held responsible for the adverse results upon you or your children.

Article 3

While all immunization laws have exceptions you can use, the wording in each state differs, and you must know the exact wording for your state to make the proper request of waiver. This information can be obtained in one of two ways.

1. Go to the reference section of your local library- look in the State Statute Revised Law Book under Public Health Law or Communicable Disease sections. The list of immunization requirements will appear first and then the exemptions will be given. Usually one or two provisions will be listed: either on religious or medical grounds or both.

2. You may call or write your state representative and ask for a copy of the immunization laws in your state. Making this available is part of his job, and it will be sent promptly.

Rule No. 3: Know your own state law so that you can conform to its exact requirements for exemption.

Article 4

There are two basic reasons for exception—medical or religious. Which one you choose will often depend upon the wording of the law in your state and your personal convictions.

We shall discuss medical exemption first. While laws do vary, nearly all states require that a note or certificate of waiver be submitted by a physician licensed in the state of residence. In some areas where states are small and people continually travel from one to another for business, a statement from a physician in a contiguous state will be accepted.

In this letter, it is usually necessary to state the reason for the requested waiver and the length of time it should extend. Many laws limit all such letters to a school year and must be renewed each fall.

The two most valid reasons for medical waiver are "the fear of allergic reaction in a sensitive child" and "to prevent possible damage to a weakened immune system." Both of these can occur in a child who has been immunized, and since no one but the physician and the parent will be held responsible for their consequences, it is up to them to protect the child.

It is possible that some states may require the letter from an M.D. or D.O., but many will allow an exemption letter from a chiropractor if it is courteously and properly written, as outlined above.

Rule No. 4: Medical waivers are always valid but must be written to fit each state law and often need to be renewed annually.

Article 5

The foregoing may work for school exemptions, but are there any such waivers in the Armed Forces? Yes. All branches of the Service provide "immunization waivers."

Again, if they did not, you could sue them for millions of dollars if a reaction occurred from their immunizations. Because of these waiver provisions, you become responsible if you react.

When you first sign up or enlist, you must state your objection to the vaccinations and tell whether it is "religious conscience" or medical reasons, such as allergies or a low tolerance to medication of any kind. If you do not show objection at this time, you have given the military the right to do what they will with you.

If there is any difficulty, the same rules apply here as in the school program. Never forget, even though you may be in the Service, no one has the right to immunize you against your will. You do not give up your constitutional rights when you join the Armed Forces.

Rule No. 5: The rules that govern school vaccination exemption also apply to the military. Never let anyone tell you otherwise. They do not know, or are hiding, the facts of the law.

Article 6

What about international travel? May I go around the world without vaccination?

The World Health Organization (WHO) in Geneva grants American visitors the right to REFUSE shots when traveling internationally. However, if an area you wish to enter is infected, you may be detained until the public health servant gives you the "go" (at his discretion).

Thousands travel world-wide each year without shots, so you may if that is your choice. Many of our co-workers have traveled over much of the world and have never taken any immunizations, nor were they ever detained.

It would be wise to request a copy of Foreign Rules and Regulations, Part 71, Title 42, on immunization when you receive your passport. Never forget the basic rule, "No one will vaccinate you against your will because by doing so they assume full responsibility for the consequences both legal and medical."

Rule No. 6: You may travel wherever you wish in the world without vaccination. The worst that can happen is that in very rare circumstances you may be detained temporarily.

Some Important Details

The above seven articles constitute all the basic rules. However, there are many important little "tricks of the trade" to having your legal requests honored. These will now be discussed.

While waivers and exemptions are written into all laws on immunization, most public health officials, doctors, and especially school officials are loathe to discuss their existence when questioned, and rarely, to our knowledge, volunteer such information.

A top Philadelphia school official was heard on the radio making the unequivocal statement, "NO SHOTS, NO SCHOOL."

This statement is, of course, completely counter to state law, with which presumably he is familiar. Such unwarranted dogmatism is common in the people you will encounter. Once the end of their legitimate authority has been reached, they will use their next most powerful weapon—INTIMIDATION.

They will threaten to keep your child out of school, take him from you, or send you to jail. These are all idle threats because they can do none of these things if you follow our simple instructions.

The basic rules have been given to you, but there are a few important details to be considered if the officials start on this course of unlawful intimidation.

1. You must send a letter to the school to inform the education officials of your stand. A phone call is not legal. It can be a note from your doctor, minister, or a notarized letter from you stating your sincere objections to the immunization. If you do not do this and fail to have your child immunized, it could be construed as negligence on your part and in some states, there is a possibility of legal action against you.

2. If the school should refuse to honor your letter, request that they give you a statement in writing outlining their reasons for refusal. If they won't, their refusal is legally invalid, and your letter stands; they must enroll your child. If they do (they rarely will) they take the risk of incriminating themselves, especially if they are acting contrary (as is common) to what is specified in the law concerning your rights for exemption. Remember they are on tenuous ground, not you. They are your servants; you are not their servant. If worst comes to worst and you have a very knowledgeable official who writes you a refusal and states accurately the lawful reasons for refusal, he will also in a negative way tell you what the accepted exemptions are, and then you can go about meeting them, by one of the routes suggested in this handout.

3. Child neglect is the one legal point you want to avoid at all costs. No legal parent or guardian can be charged with neglect unless he shows complete lack of concern or action to be more informed. Stripped of legal jargon, this simply means that if you can show that you have investigated the situation, have come to a specific decision concerning immunizations, and have informed the authorities of the same, no neglect charge can be brought. Neglect can be brought only when it can be shown that you have failed to have your children immunized, not out of respect for their medical or spiritual integrity, but only because you were too concerned with other matters.

4. At times there may be a question of whether you have given or withdrawn legal consent. Legal consent is dependent upon being properly informed on both the advantages and the risks in any choice or decision you make. In other words, if a

physician were to tell you that vaccination is perfectly safe and effective to obtain your consent, such consent would not be legal because he lied and you have not been properly informed. Conversely, it could be argued that non-consent is not legal if you are not fully informed about the risks and advantages of immunizations.

5. What do I do if everyone refuses to give me a waiver?

This would be an extremely rare circumstance. But should it happen, you are not left without resources. Here is where we pull out one of our big guns. Send notarized letters by certified mail to the vaccine laboratory which makes the shot (ask your doctor for the address), to the doctor who is to administer the shot, to your school principal, to the school board, and to your local health department.

In these letters make it clear that since they have refused to give you a duly requested waiver, you can no longer be held responsible for what may happen to your child if they force these shots upon him. You then state that you will allow immunization if each will present you with a written signed guarantee of safety and effectiveness of the vaccine and that they will consent to assume full responsibility for any and all adverse reactions that your child may develop from the required shots. Of course, none will give you such a guarantee. They cannot do so because all vaccines are considered potentially highly toxic. We have yet to hear of an instance of further harassment of parents after such letters have been sent.

That's about all that is needed to obtain the necessary exemptions for your children. All that has been said in this last section (1 to 5) is also applicable to the military and international travel, if required.

Potpourri of Ammunition

"As long as each individual who opposes vaccines has sincere objections, states them in writing, and signs his name—it is considered legal and proper action and must therefore be honored."

"Since many medical controversies exist surrounding immunization, drugs, and various other medications, it mandates that each individual have the right to control his own decisions and freedom of choice; anything less would be contrary to the constitutional laws that protect the citizens' rights."

"When you deal with school officials and lawyers, you are playing with legal terminology—move the wrong words around and you get hung." The terminology used in this booklet has worked before and should work again.

"It is important to state your objections in such a way that it complies with your state's exemption provisions. They must then accept your request; if they do not, they are breaking their own law." That is why it is absolutely essential that you know your own state law word for word before submitting your objection.

"According to CDC (the federal Communicable Disease Center in Atlanta, Georgia), physicians are required to first inform their patients of the risks involved before they consent to vaccines." If they do not do so, it is prima facie evidence of deceit or negligence on the part of the physician.

This regulation by the federal government would also seem to assume that the patient has the right to refuse if he feels that the risks are too great. If this is so, is not the federal government on record as supporting voluntary immunization and, by obvious implication, against state-enforced compulsory immunization?

Should you ever have to go to court, or what is more likely, to appear before a "kangaroo" court of school and health department officials, here is some class A evidence you might find useful to mention.

- No vaccine carries any guarantee of protection from the laboratory that produced it or the doctor who administered it.
- The U.S. military allows no-nonsense "immunizations waivers."
- There is **NO FEDERAL LAW** on immunizations. They don't dare. Their lawyers know the consequences.
- Your rights have been infringed upon by officials attempting to use force against your will.

Most state officials like a nice, stress-free job. When you send in your objections and refuse to fit their ordered world by not having your children immunized, you make waves.

This rocks their quiet existence, and there are only two ways their life can become orderly again: either by forcing you to their will or acquiescing to yours. What you must do to obtain an early waiver is to make the latter the easiest path for them.

At first, however, an attempt will usually be made to bend you to their will by some form of intimidation. Many uninformed parents give in to this tack, and so it is tried again and again.

If you are adequately informed, as a reader of this publication should be, you will let the officials know in no uncertain terms that you understand your rights under the law and will not stand for any such shilly-shallying. Invariably, once they discover you are adamant and acquainted with the state law, your waiver will be rapidly forthcoming.

An Acknowledgment

The greatest part of the material on the first four pages is taken from the work of Mrs. Grace Girdwain, of Burbank, Illinois. Our staff has rearranged and edited the information, but we wish the full credit for its existence to go to this courageous woman who has for twelve years worked arduously, without compensation, to help her fellow Americans obtain their legal rights.

The following is an example of the state of Illinois law (where I live) relating to immunizations. Illinois, like most states, has no philosophical objection, but does have a religious one.

Illinois Administrative Code Title 77: Public Health
Chapter I: Department of Public Health
Subchapter i: Maternal and Child Health
Part 665 Child Health Examination Code
Subpart E: Exceptions

Section 665.510 Objection of Parent or Legal Guardian

Parent or legal guardian of a student may object to health examinations, immunizations, vision, and hearing screening tests, and dental health examinations for their children on religious grounds. If a religious objection is made, a written and signed statement from the parent or legal guardian detailing such objections must be presented to the local school authority.

General philosophical or moral reluctance to allow physical examinations, immunizations, vision and hearing screening, and dental examinations will not provide a sufficient basis for an exception to statutory requirements.

The parent or legal guardian must be informed by the local school authority of measles outbreak control exclusion procedures per IDPH rules. The Control of Communicable Diseases (77 Ill. Adm. Code 690) at the time such objection is presented.

Section 665.520 Medical Objections

a) Any medical objections to an immunization must be:
1) Made by a physician licensed to practice medicine in all its branches indicating what the medical condition is.
2) Endorsed and signed by the physician on the certificate of child health examination and placed on file in the child's permanent record.

b) Should the condition of the child later permit immunization, this requirement will then have to be met. Parents or legal guardians must be informed of measles outbreak control exclusion procedures when such objection is presented per Section 665.510.

APPENDIX B
Recommended Ingredients and Products Locator

Some of the foods and health products recommended in this book, can be found in health food stores. If you want further insight on the best forms and brands of these foods and products, you can consult the following lists.

The first list contains all the foods and other health products and services that I have researched extensively, that are typically more difficult to find in stores, and that I offer through the "Most Popular Products" section of Mercola.com.

The second list contains some specific foods and kitchen equipment that you can order direct from the suppliers or other online stores.

**For the most updated products go to
takecontrolof yourhealth.com/resources**

Krill Oil

Krill Oil has more health-promoting antioxidants and omega-3 oils than fish oil. As a matter of fact, it has over 47 times the antioxidant value of fish oil which helps prevent the perishable omega-3 from becoming rancid. Not only that, but there's no aftertaste.

APPENDIX B

Cocoa Cassava Bars

Finally—a health-smart snack bar. These are an amazing alternative to the typical energy bars currently out on the market that are loaded with less-than-optimal ingredients like sugars, soy protein and artificial sweeteners. Not only are they healthy for you, they also taste great! Even kids love eating them. Cocoa Cassava Bars work well as a pick-me-up, or as a healthy snack.

Radical Fruits

Radical Fruits contains a blend of 10 antioxidant-rich fruits and alkalizing minerals which form a potent synergistic combination with a very high ORAC value. (ORAC scores are used to measure antioxidant activity.) It also has polyphenolic bioflavonoids including resveratrol which supports good overall health as it helps your body reduce free radicals. Radical Fruits promotes cardiovascular and immune function and allows you to obtain the necessary nutrients from fruit—even out of season.

FucoThin

FucoThin is a natural, whole food based supplement made with proprietary concentration of marine-derived brown seaweed and pomagranate seed oil, for a patent-pending formula that provides thermogenic support to help maximize your weight control efforts. FucoThin supports the metabolism or breakdown of fat in white adipose tissue, including belly fat, without stimulating the central nervous system.

Coconut Oil, Virgin and Organic

Virgin coconut oil is highly recommended for your cooking, and has a wide range of proven health benefits. But quality can vary widely among brands, so you have to know what you are looking for. Fresh Shores and Garden of Life brand coconut oils meet all the necessary requirements, including certified organic, non-GMO, no "copra" or dried coconuts used, and no hydrogenation.

Cookware—5 Piece Enameled Cast Iron

Don't endanger your family's health with potentially toxic pots and pans, including Teflon, aluminum, stainless steel, and copper. Now you can cook healthy and delicious meals at home with this gorgeous updated cast iron cookware. This set includes a 5 quart oval casserole with lid, 2 quart saucepan with lid, and 10 inch fry pan. This beautiful and affordable set comes with a limited lifetime warranty.

Coconut Flour

Replace coconut flour with your desserts and eat them guilt-free! Coconut flour is free of glutens and low in digestible carbohydrates. It promotes a healthy heart and immune system. Coconut flour is packed with fiber, so you'll feel full faster. It's a great way to help control your health and manage your weight.

Full Spectrum Light Bulbs

Way Healthier has created a healthy way to receive many of the benefits of sunshine during the short days of winter and when it is cloudy. The full spectrum light bulbs accurately mimic the midday sun. They're also only 20 or 30 watts and put out the same amount of light as a 100 watt light bulb. So not only will they help you get healthier, but they'll save you money too and keep the environment greener!

Himalayan Salt

It comes in two forms—cooking salt and in bath crystals. Regular table salt contains little to no value and can actually contribute to cellulite, rheumatism, arthritis, and kidney and gall stones. Himalayan Salt can help restore your balance and can be used in too many ways to mention here! Look at my website for more information.

Air Purifier

Way Healthier's Home Air Purifier is a great choice for anyone who suffers from allergies triggered by allergens or the person with a high level of unwanted chemicals in their house. It is entirely noiseless, reduces particle pollution, and will save you money (there are no replacement filters needed). Plus, it's a great value.

Juicer, Omega 8003 and 8005 Models

I have done an extensive evaluation of juicers and found that the Omega 8003 and 8005 Juicers are the clear winners in terms of their multiple uses, durability, ease of use and cleaning, and value. You can find an extensive juicer evaluation chart comparing the various juicers at Mercolo.com as well.

Kefir Starter and Culture Starter

Traditionally fermented foods are an essential part of every healthy diet, and the Kefir Starter and Culture Starter available here an exceptionally high-quality way to make your own fermented foods very quickly and inexpensively. Kefir is an ancient – and still one of nature's most powerful and delicious – health foods, and the Kefir Starter enables very easy preparation. The Culture Starter, meanwhile, is a simple way to make your vegetables into very healthy and delicious traditional fermented foods.

Salmon, Wild Red Alaskan and Toxin-Free

This Vital Choice brand of salmon is the *only* fish I have found, through independent laboratory testing we had performed on the fish, to be free from harmful mercury, PCBs and other toxins. It is a premier source of omega-3 with EHA and DPA fatty acids, is high in antioxidants, and is free of antibiotics, pesticides, synthetic coloring agents, growth hormones and GMOs. It also tastes absolutely incredible!

Foods—Other Suppliers

Herbs and Seasonings, Organic
Herbal Advantage, Inc., 1-800-753-9199
www.herbaladvantage.com

Milk and Cream, Raw
Go to www.realmilk.com to find out if there are cow-share programs in your area

Nuts and Seeds, Raw and Organic
Jaffe Brothers Natural Foods, 1-760-749-1133, www.organicfruit-sandnuts.com

Spike®/ Salt-Free Spike
Famous all-purpose vegetable seasoning
Modern Products, 800-877-8935, www.modernfearn.com or in most grocery stores

Spouting Seeds, Organic
Complete line of organic seeds
The Sproutpeople, 877-777-6887, www.sproutpeople.com

Stevia
Non-carb, non-glycemic, non-synthetic, alternative sweetener
Available in liquid concentrate and baking powder
Body Ecology, 800-511-2660, bodyecologydiet.com

Kitchen Equipment – Other Suppliers

Food Dehydrators
Excalibur Dehydrator®
Excalibur Products, 1-800-875-4254, www.excaliburdehydrator.com

Juicers
See www.takecontrolofyourhealth.com/kitchen

Spiral SlicerTM
Manual slicer & processor for creating pasta from vegetables
see www.takecontrolofyourhealth.com/kitchen

Sprouters
Sprouting equipment and seeds
The Sproutpeople, 1-877-777-6887, www.sproutpeople.com

Recommended Resources and Further Reading

Books

Sweet Deception—Why Splenda, NutraSweet and the FDA May Be Hazardous to Your Health

Authors: Dr. Joseph Mercola, Dr. Kendra Degen Pearsall

Perhaps you thought you'd been making a healthier choice by substituting those friendly little blue, pink and yellow packets for sugar (particularly if you're a dieter with a sweet tooth). Tragically, the truth is this: artificial sweeteners such as Splenda and Nutrasweet are NOT healthy—or safe.

Venture with me, if you dare, into the dark heart and soul of the giant food and drug corporations ... and your own government.

Discover the inside story. See how you've been deceived about the truth behind artificial sweeteners like aspartame and sucralose—for greed, for profit . . . and at the expense of your own health.

Generation XL

Authors: Dr. Joseph Mercola and Dr. Ben Lerner

There is a worldwide obesity epidemic and this book addresses the reasons why this has occurred, but more importantly offers simple practical strategies that can be easily implemented so your child is spared the ravages and harm that obesity causes.

The Metabolic Typing Diet: Customize Your Diet to Your Own Unique Body Chemistry

Authors: William L. Wolcott, with Trish Fahey

This book is the foundation of our Nutritional Typing Program. Our team has revised, simplified and improved the concepts to make it work even better for you. This is a good book to understand nutrional typing roots.

Nutrition and Physical Degeneration

Author: Dr. Weston Price

I often my refer patients to this wonderful resource. This is a pioneering work in natural health and simply a must-read if you are interested in the foundational truths of nutrition. Dr. Westin Price was one of the most prominent dentists at the turn of the century and wondered why so many children were getting cavities. He realized that it was the introduction of processed foods. So he traveled the world and documented the connection between processed foods and ill health, and the principles he developed still largely hold true today.

The Whole Soy Story
Author: Dr. Kaayla Daniel

This extensively researched and compelling read dispels the myths that soybeans are a major "health food" and pinpoints why they can lead to health challenges instead.

Pace: Rediscover Your Native Fitness
Author: Al Sears, M.D.

This book exposes the myths and misconceptions about health, aging and fitness.

Remember Wholeness: A Personal Handbook for Thriving in the 21st Century
Author: Carol Tuttle

A simple and profound approach to creating the life you want and deserve.

Video and Audio Resources

Look for these video and audio health resources in the "Recommended Products" section of Mercola.com.

EFT Training Course

EFT is profoundly effective emotional and mental healing approach that is based on the principles of energy medicine. I have taught it to the patients in my clinic for years, and they have experienced truly incredible and permanent results with it.

Because EFT can help with everything (negative emotions, physical problems—it can even help you lower your golf score!) I think everyone can benefit from taking Gary Craig's "The EFT Course." The EFT Course contains over 13 hours of video instruction.

To learn more please visit www.mercola.com/eft

Carol Tuttle Healing Center

    1. "Master Energy Therapist" Carol Tuttle is a widely respected expert in the areas of Energy Psychology and Energy Medicine. Carol has produced many informational products that can help you identify the blocks and patterns that are keeping you from reaching your life potential and to help you achieve what you want in life such as weight loss and financial abundance.

To learn more visit www.mercola.com/Tuttle

Newsletters & Websites

Dr. Mercola's "eHealthy News You Can Use"
Subscribe at Mercola.com

My free thrice-weekly newsletter reaching one million subscribers as of this writing, provides you with the most important and timely health news and information that can help you take control of your health and will also warn you of the deception and misinformation that is so prevalent in the health field.

Mercola.com

My website, with over 100,000 pages of useful articles and information on virtually any health topic you may be interested in, is now the world's most visited natural health website. Whenever you have a question about any health or dietary topic, simply go to Mercola.com and enter the phrase in the powerful—and free—search engine.

ENLITA.COM

ENLITA™ is an organization founded by Dr. Kendra Pearsall and Dr. Joseph Mercola to provide you with online education programs in specific areas of health and wellness. Our first program will focus on natural and holistic weight loss. If you want to discover how to attain your ideal weight with natural lifestyle changes, go to ENLITA.COM today.

The Weston A. Price Foundation

www.westonaprice.org

The Weston A. Price Foundation

A nonprofit organization founded in 1999. Their goals are to provide accurate information on nutrition and human health, including the vital importance of animal fats in the diet, and to provide the resources and information necessary to help people transition to a natural way of eating.

The Price-Pottenger Nutrition Foundation

www.price-pottenger.org

The Price-Pottenger Nutrition Foundation (PPNF) is another nonprofit organization whose main goal is to educate the public about the findings of Dr. Weston A. Price. They focus on disseminating the information gathered and researched by one of Price's better-known colleagues, Dr. Francis Pottenger. The discoveries of these two men have helped to form the basis of what we believe to be a truly healthy die.

Center for Science in the Public Interest

www.cspinet.org

Center for Science in the Public Interest (CSPI) was established in 1971 as a national advocate for proper nutrition, food safety, alcohol policy, and sound scientific research. They have effected many positive health changes in the food industry.

Some of CSPI's past accomplishments include the following:

- A new federal law enacted that sets standards for health claims on food labels and provides full and clear nutrition information on nearly all packaged foods (including the labeling of trans-fat per serving)

- Millions of Americans changed their food choices at popular restaurants thanks to CSPI's widely publicized studies on the nutritional value of restaurants meals; thousands of restaurants have added healthier options to their menus.

- Major fast-food chains have begun introducing healthier foods

- Scores of deceptive ads by companies such as McDonald's, Kraft, and Campbell's Soup have been stopped

Organic Consumers Association

www.organicconsumers.org

Organic Consumers Association (OCA) is an on-line and grass-roots non-profit public interest organization campaigning for health, justice, and sustainability. The OCA deals with crucial issues of food safety, industrial agriculture, genetic engineering, children's health, corporate accountability, Fair trade, environmental sustainability and other key topics.

Acres USA

www.acresusa.com

Acres USA is dedicated to educating consumers and farmers about sustainable agriculture and food development practices, while providing an insider's view on the misguided practices of chemical farming. They provide an excellent magazine, online articles, and more.

American Association for Health Freedom (AAHF)

www.healthfreedom.net

AAHF was founded in 1992 in direct response to the problems faced by health care practitioners and consumers in the United States. AAHF works as an advocate to restore the medical freedoms that have been threatened by the U.S. Food and Drug Administration, the allopathic medical community, insurance companies, and state medical boards around the United States.

Environmental Working Group (EWG)

www.ewg.org

EWG specializes in environmental investigations. They have a team of scientists, engineers, policy experts, lawyers, and computer programmers who examine data from a variety of sources to expose threats to your health and the environment, and to find solutions.

www.realmilk.com

A fantastic resource by The Weston A. Price Foundation providing everything you need to know about healthy raw milk. Includes detail on why raw milk is so nutritious, if its sales are legal in your regions, and where specifically to find cowshare programs or suppliers in your area.

Health Science Institute

www.hsibaltimore.com

The mission of the Health Science Institute, including their excellent newsletter, is to keep you informed of smart preventive choices that will help you take control of your health.

Union of Concerned Scientists

www.ucsusa.org

Union of Concerned Scientists is the leading science based nonprofit working for health environment and a safe world. UCS combines independent scientific research and action to develop innovative, practical solution and to secure responsible changes in government policy, corporate practices and consumer choices.

APPENDIX C
Simple Principles to Know if Your Diet Works for You

A right diet is one that gives you lasting energy throughout the day, no indigestion, 2–3 bowel movements per day, and is composed mostly of natural, unprocessed foods. Also, good skin conditions and white eyes are a sign that your diet is working for you. Poor skin, rings or bags under your eyes, and discoloration of your eyes are a tell-tale sign that your diet may not be right for you.

The purpose of your meal is to leave you feeling satiated and comfortable (no longer hungry). It is not natural to stuff your stomach until you are so full you can barely move. Most Westerners are raised to eat like this, and it's one of the causes of the obesity epidemic we face. So, try to get used to eating smaller portions.

- If in doubt, leave it out. If you're not sure if something is bad for you, it probably is. If you can, use your willpower and resist. Have an extra portion of fruit or salad instead.

- Stay away from junk food snacks and processed foods.

- Do not regularly consume sugary desserts. Reserve them for special occasions only.

- Eat out less and avoid fast food. This means bring your lunch to work.

- Never drink soda of any kind.

- If you can, eat your lunch outside as well so you can relax, enjoy nature, and get some sunshine to boost your energy and mood. It takes a little more effort, but it's worth it.

Lots of colors and variety: your plate should look like a tropical rainbow of different fruits, vegetables, legumes, and nuts.

ABOUT THE AUTHORS

About the Authors:

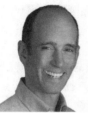

Dr. Joseph Mercola is the founder of Mercola.com, the world's most visited natural health website. He is also the author of the 2006 best selling *Sweet Deception* and two *New York Times* bestsellers, *The Great Bird Flu Hoax*, and *The No-Grain Diet*.

As an osteopathic physician, Dr. Mercola first trained in conventional medicine and later received extensive training in natural medicine. He graduated medical school in 1982 at Midwestern University in Chicago. He has served as Chairman of the Department of Family Practice at St. Alexius Hospital in Illinois for five years and has been interviewed and profiled extensively for his health and dietary expertise, including the *New York Times*, *Wall Street Journal*, *Time Magazine*, ABC's *World News Tonight*, CBS, ABC, NBC, Fox TV and CNN.

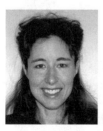

Dr. Kendra Pearsall is a Naturopathic Physician who has specialized in natural weight loss ever since she graduated from Southwest College of Naturopathic Medicine in Tempe, Arizona in 2001. She is the co-author of *Sweet Deception* and *Dr. Mercola's Take Control Of Your Health* and is the medical editor of *The Hormone Handbook*. Pearsall's mission is to teach people how to achieve permanent weight loss through lifestyle changes with her weight loss website: **ENLITA.com**. Pearsall's interests include researching health, politics and religion, world travel, spending time in nature, and creating a future health resort.

About The Contributing Writers

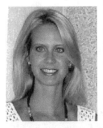

Rachael Droege is the former managing editor of Mercola.com and a current regular contributor. She is also a freelance natural health writer and editor, with specialties in natural living, nutrition, spirituality, and holistic medicine. Her works have appeared in numerous magazines, Web sites and newsletters. Rachael is also an avid creative writer and poet, with a passion to inspire others to live well and enjoy life.

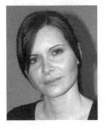

Darcy Langdon has been in the wellness-beauty field for ten years. Her landmark of *beauty coming from within* has inspired her to merge her skills as an esthetician and nutritionist. Darcy believes that beauty must begin as an inner-transformation, with an emphasis on nourishing the body with healing foods, emotional healing and prioritizing non-toxic personal care products as a foundation for health. Darcy has been a student of Dr. Mercola's since 2000 and a health consultant for the Optimal Wellness center since 2002.

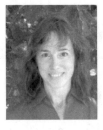

Colleen Huber, NMD is a Naturopathic Medical Doctor and primary care physician. She completed her medical training at Southwest College of Naturopathic Medicine in Tempe, Arizona, Southwest Naturopathic Medical Center in Scottsdale, AZ, and has her private practice in Tempe. Her website www.naturopathyworks.com introduces naturopathic medicine to the layperson and provides references to the abundant medical literature demonstrating that natural medicine does work. She has written for the world's largest health site, www.Mercola.com, on nutrition topics. Her original research on migraines has appeared in *Lancet* and *Headache Quarterly*, and was reported in *The Washington Post*.

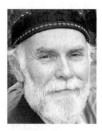

Dr. Isaac Golden, is a practicing homeopath and an acknowledged world authority on the safety and effectiveness of homeopathic immunization (or homoeoprophylaxis). He has conducted over 20 years of research into homoeoprophylaxis, including the world's largest, long-term trial of the method, which has shown it to be safe, and comparably effective to vaccination. He is the author of *Vaccination & Homoeoprophylaxis? A Review of Risks and Alternatives, 6th edition,* which fully explains his 5 year immunisation program, and makes a balanced comparison between the safety and effectiveness of vaccination and the homoeopathic alternative. People who are interested Dr. Golden's research into his long-term immunisation program, should visit his web site www.homstudy.net .

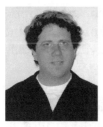

Ry Herman is a writer and editor with a lifelong interest in science, health, and nutrition. He was the editor of, and a contributor to, Dr. Mercola's previous books, *Sweet Deception* and *The Great Bird Flu Hoax,* and for the past two years, he has edited the Mercola.com thrice-weekly online newsletter. Currently, he is collaborating with Dr. Mercola on the upcoming book, *Dark Deception,* an in-depth examination of vitamin D, sunlight, and health. Ry is also an award-winning playwright, and his plays have been produced throughout the U.S. and internationally.

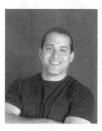

Ryan Lee is the most in-demand fitness expert in the world. He has helped over 100,000 get fit, lose weight and improve their sports performance through his training programs, workshops, products, websites and sold out seminars. He's a training advisor to *Men's Fitness* and has been featured in media outlets such as *USA Today, NY Times, Wall Street Journal, Men's Journal, Personal Fitness Professional, Golf Illustrated* and many more.

Download 15 FREE workouts by Ryan by visiting http://quatro-fitness.com

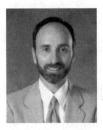

Jeffrey M. Smith is a widely popular and authoritative spokesperson on the risks of Genetically Modified Organisms (GMOs). He has counseled dozens of world leaders from every continent, changed the course of government policies, and is now orchestrating a shift in public opinion through his programs at the Institute for Responsible Technology. He has spoken in 25 countries and has been quoted in media across the globe including, *The New York Times*, *Washington Post*, *BBC World Service*, and *Nature*.

A masterful storyteller, his hard-to-put-down accounts of industry manipulation and political collusion promoted his first book, *Seeds of Deception*, into the world's bestseller on GMOs. His just-released new book, *Genetic Roulette: The documented health risks of genetically engineered foods*, represents a two-year collaboration with more than 30 scientists. He is the producer of the docu-video series, *The GMO Trilogy*, and writes an internationally syndicated column, Spilling the Beans. He lives with his wife in Iowa, surrounded by genetically modified soy and corn.

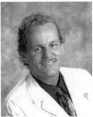

Al Sears, MD is a member of the American Academy of Anti-Aging Medicine and is Board Certified in Anti-Aging Medicine. As a pioneer in this new field of medicine, he is an avid researcher and sought after lecturer to thousands of doctors and health enthusiasts.

He is a member of the American College of Sports Medicine and the National Youth Sports Coaches Association. As well as being a sports and fitness coach and a lifelong advocate of exercise programs, Dr. Sears is an ACE certified fitness trainer. He publishes a monthly newsletter—*Health Confidential*—addressing the issues of aging, nutrition and sexual health for men and women, and a weekly e-letter called *Doctor's House*.

ABOUT THE AUTHORS

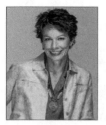 Carol Tuttle is an energy psychologist, best-selling author, and an incredibly successful speaker. She has appeared on hundreds of radio shows and made numerous local and national television appearances. She and her husband, Jon, reside in Salt Lake City, UT and utilize these energy clearing techniques in their everyday lives with their 5 children. Carol's best-selling book, *Remembering Wholeness*, and her other products have helped transform the lives of hundreds of thousand of people. In addition, she has launched *The Carol Tuttle Healing Center*, an interactive website utilizing these techniques for clearing literally hundreds of issues. For more information go to www.mercola.com/Tuttle